CMAA Certification Study Guide

Medical Administrative Assistant

Certification Prep

Key Points Exam Prep Team

CMAA Certification Study Guide

Medical Administrative Assistant Certification Prep

Copyright © 2015 by Key Points Exam Prep Team

All rights reserved. No part of this book may be reproduced or transmitted in any form or by any means without written permission from the author.

ISBN-13: 978-1505781137

ISBN-10: 1505781132

Printed in the United States of America.

Purchase at www.djngbooks.org

Dedication

To all Medical Administrative Assistant Students

Test Taking Strategies

1. Set goals for yourself: 30 days before your exam, set the goal of finishing one module per day. If you keep to this goal and accomplish it day after day, you will have 4 days still open before your exam day. Use 3 days to touch any areas you feel you need to still practice more. On the last day before your exam, sleep very well, relax, take out time for yourself and let your brain be ready for your test the next day.

2. Discipline yourself for study: Do not study at home, unless you do not have things to distract you. If you cannot refrain yourself from turning on the TV, or checking the internet, or checking your text messages, go to the library, and leave your phone in your trunk! All those text messages and emails can wait till you finish your study. There is a flow of study that comes when you concentrate to internalize information. The brain is somewhat prepared, knowing that study time has come. I have experienced it over and over whenever I am serious about studying. I have also experienced the breakage in the process that comes when this study time is full of distractions. It seems to me that the brain becomes confused as to if you really want to study or not, and so retracts. Devoting ample time to study without distraction is a key to passing any major exam.

3. Identify areas of weakness: If you are not competent yet on medical terminology, spend more time on studying it; If filing is the problem, Practice! Practice!! Practice!!!

4. Listen in class: It is very important to listen to the teacher and listen to her examples and illustrations. Understanding the topic the first time it is taught in class is very vital to further studies. I have seen students who are so busy searching their textbooks for information when I am teaching in class. Those are the students who are filled with anxiety when exam approaches because they feel they have not learnt anything. How would you learn when you did not pay attention in class? It is not all the information in the textbook that you need to pass your exam. Actually, some information in some textbooks are meant to complete the pages. That is why you need to pay attention in class so as to know where to concentrate on your extra study. You may spend more hours studying while someone else spends less hours studying the right things because they have a guided study.

5. Do not give in to exam anxiety: Excessive anxiety can make you to be disorganized and start forgetting the things you have studied. That is why I suggested earlier that you do not study the day before your exam, so as to relax. Remember that people have passed this exam before. If they could pass it the first time, you should too. This should help you to enter the exam hall with confidence.

Contents

The Medical Assistant Duties and Responsibilities
Medical Law, Medical Profession Liability
The Patient Care Partnership (Patient's Bill of Rights)
The HIPAA Patient Privacy Rule
Legal Terms
Communication
Phone Etiquette
Verbal and Nonverbal Communication
Respect Scheduling
Appointment Booking
Appointment Setting
Types of Scheduling
Scheduling New Patients
Scheduling Established Patients
Scheduling Conflicts
Letter Writing
Mail Processing Incoming Mail
Outgoing Mail
Health Insurance
Verification of Insurance Benefits
Insurance Terms
Medical Records Management
Creating a Medical Record
Filing
Indexing
Alphabetical Filing Numerical Filing Subject Filing
Tickler File
Medical Terminology

The Medical Administrative Assistant Duties and Responsibilities

The medical administrative assistant is some employed in healthcare facilities to perform non-patient care duties that in turn helps the care given to patients appear organized, manageable and profitable. They are employed to perform a wide array of duties in the offices of various health professions. These duties include telephone coverage, scheduling, maintenance of medical records, and the management of all correspondences.

The professional qualities that the Medical Administrative Assistant should possess include the following:

- Dependability
- Courtesy
- Initiative
- Interpersonal Skills

Medical Law

The medical administrative assistant is required to have a basic understanding of the legal principles which set the standard for the professional duties and limitations of the members of a medical practice.

Medical Profession Liability

The physician-patient relationship is an implied contract in which the physician is expected to assess and treat the patient with the same amount of knowledge, skill, and judgment as another physician. Under this agreement, the following rules must be followed:

- The patient is expected to compensate the physician for all services provided.
- The patient is expected to adhere to any directions or guidance provided by the physician.

☐ If the physician terminates the contract, the patient must be provided with advance notice of these intentions as well as given enough time to seek the services of another physician.

Once a physician-patient relationship has been entered, the physician must have consent to treat the patient. In most cases, the patient's implied consent is apparent through their action of seeking the services of the physician. In certain situations, the patient's informed consent is necessary, in a written form that states their understanding of the prescribed treatment as well as its accompanying risks.

In the event that a patient has not provided consent and is in need of emergency assistance, the physician or any other health care worker will be protected by the Good Samaritan Act, which states that a volunteer is not held liable for any civil damages that may occur as a result of their efforts to provide emergency care.

Communication

A. Principles of communication: For communication to be complete, there needs to be a feedback from the individual or party the message had been sent to. Do not assume that the message was sent or understood without a confirmation.

A. Important steps in communication:
 1. Message
 2. Sender
 3. Receiver
 4. Interpretation

B. Methods used in communicating:
 1. Verbal:
    a. Spoken words

2. Non-verbal:

a. Conscious and unconscious

b. Types:

    1) body language

    2) touch

c. Written

    1) labels - like red dots, armbands

    2) visual labels – name tags and uniforms

3. Electronic:

a. Devices to "create" sound of words (verbal)

b. Computers/touch pads to type words/phrases onto screen

B. Common reasons for communication breakdown and methods for correction.

    Verbal barriers

    a. Criticism

    b. Value statements

    c. Interruptions

    d. Judgment

    e. Language differences

    f. Changing subjects

    g. Excessive talking

2. Non-verbal barriers:

    a. Body language

    b. Eye contact

    c. Cultural differences

3. Physiological/aging factors:

   a. Hearing loss

   b. Vision loss

   c. Response time

   d. Medication

4. Not listening – listening is hard work (barriers).

   a. Lack of concentration:

   1) Preoccupied

   2) Distracting noises

   3) Monotone voice

   4) Negative attitude

   b. Selective hearing – is what one wants or expects to hear

   c. Emotional response to a word or situation

C. Use effective communication skills with patients and team members.

D. Be aware of non-verbal forms of communication.

E. Evaluate ability of others to understand, asking for feedback.

F. Use assertive communication such as "I" messages, giving and receiving feedback, and clarifying instructions.

G. Respect the health care team structure and lines of authority.

H. Communicating with individuals with special needs:

1. Language/cultural differences:

   a. Ask for an interpreter if the resident or family is unable to speak English or the language of the CNA.

   b. Know cultural beliefs – on word use, gestures and touching.

2. Visually impaired:

- a. Describe surroundings to a visually impaired resident.
- b. Identify self when entering resident's room.
- c. Do not touch resident until they know you are there.
- d. Explore the room with resident.
- e. Do not rearrange the room.
- f. Explain all you do.
- g. Let resident know when you have finished and are leaving the room.
- h. Keep doors open.
- i. Monitor meals.
- j. Do not speak loudly.

3. Hearing impaired:
   - a. Gain the attention of the resident, using touch as appropriate.
   - b. Determine which ear has the hearing loss.
   - c. Check to see if hearing aids are in and turned on.
   - d. Determine the percentage of hearing loss and too high/low tones.
   - e. Face the resident directly (if applicable).
     1) Do not block your mouth or chew gum.
     2) Reduce/eliminate background noise and other distractions.
     3) Stand or sit on the side of the better ear.
   - f. Speak slowly, directly, and clearly when addressing a hearing-impaired resident. Do not speak loudly
   - g. Use short sentences and simple words.
   - h. Repeat and rephrase statements as needed.

The HIPAA Patient Privacy Rule

This rule establishes regulations for the use and disclosure of protected health information and mandates that all patients be provided a copy of privacy policies when treated in a doctor's office or when admitted to any health care facility. Also, patient information cannot be shared with anyone not directly involved in their care. Examples of HIPAA violation include discussing patient information with:

   a. Healthcare worker's family members
   b. Co-workers that are not involved in patient's care
   c. Friends of healthcare worker
   d. Friends of patient

Legal Terms

Abandonment : The discontinuation of medical care without proper notice

Arbitration: The usage of an impartial third party for the hearing and determination of a dispute

Battery: The unlawful use of force or violence

Negligence : The failure to provide the necessary care that is required for a person's situation

Statues: Laws enacted by the legislative branch of a government

Communication

Phone Etiquette

Since the Medical Administrative Assistant is responsible for answering telephone calls, it is imperative to have solid communication skills.

The following steps will ensure proper telephone etiquette:

☐ Answer the telephone promptly and kindly.

☐ Be sure to properly speak into the phone.

- Be sure to give the caller your undivided attention.
- Speak clearly and distinctly.
- Always be courteous.
- Be sure to ask the caller's permission before placing them on hold.
- Never allow an angry or aggressive caller to upset you; remain calm and composed.

Verbal and Nonverbal Communication

Verbal communication is the use of the language or the actual words spoken. Some of the key components of verbal communication are sound, words, speaking, and language. Nonverbal communication is the use of eye contact, body language, facial expression, or symbolic expressions to communicate a message.

Respect

Respect is essential in the process of communication with coworkers, patients, and visitors. The following steps will help to create a comfortable environment:

- Refrain from making jokes or negative remarks that demean the abilities, skills, or aspects of co-workers
- Be patient and respectful when speaking with a caller that does not speak English clearly Scheduling

Appointment Books

The medical administrative should consider the following characteristics when selecting an appointment book:

- It's size in consideration of the amount of desk space available
- It's ability to accommodate the number of appointments made
- Comfort for writing
- Adequate space for all details necessary

In this electronic era, many medical offices are resorting to computerized booking.

Appointment Setting

Advance preparation is necessary to enable the medical administrative to schedule patients both accurately and efficiently. One method of advance preparation is the usage of the matrix. The following information should be marked in the appointment book in advance:

- Times the physician is not available to see patients
- Hospital rounds, meetings
- Physician's days off, holidays, lunch/dinner breaks etc.

Types of Scheduling

Wave scheduling: A certain number of patients are scheduled to arrive at the same time and the patients are seen in the order in which they arrive

Modified wave scheduling: Small groups of patients are scheduled at intervals throughout the hour

Double Booking: Scheduling two patients to see the physician at the same time

Scheduling New Patients

The Medical Administrative Assistant should do the following when scheduling a new patient:

- Obtain and verify general information
- Gather appropriate information regarding a patient referral
- Determine the patient's chief complaint
- Make the patient aware of the various dates and times they are available to come in
- Enter the appropriate time for the appointment
- Determine the proper financial arrangements for the patient's appointment
- Provide directions as needed
- Verify information

Scheduling Established Patients

The Medical Administrative Assistant should do the following when scheduling an established patient:

- Gather the appropriate information in order to properly identify the patient
- Ask the reason for the patient's request for an appointment
- Determine which member of the practice they would like to see, if necessary
- Provide the patient with two options for the date and time they will be able to come in
- Enter the appropriate time for the appointment
- Verify information
- Provide patient with appointment card if necessary

Scheduling Conflicts

Conflict Resolution

Late Patients Advise the patient to arrive 30 minutes before their scheduled time.

Emergency Calls Arrangements should be made for the patient to be seen the same day.

Cancelled Appointments

Make sure the original appointment time is properly removed, then schedule the new appointment.

Unscheduled Patients

Accommodate the patient as best as possible; ensure that the patient is aware that making an appointment is the most effective way to receive care.

Failed Appointments Note the absence on the patient's medical chart as well as the appointment book and attempt to reschedule

Delayed Patient Wait Time

Briefly explain the reason for delay, and provide the patient with the option to reschedule.

Mail Processing

Incoming Mail

The Medical Administrative Assistant is responsible to process the following items which come in the mail:

- General correspondence
- Payments
- Bills
- Reports

Also, she/he ensures that outgoing mails are processed.

Health Insurance

Verification of Insurance Benefits

The Medical Administrative Assistant should take the following steps in order to verify a patient's insurance benefits:

- When the patient requests an appointment, identify the type of insurance or the managed care plan that the patient is eligible for.
- Upon the patient's arrival, make copies of both sides of the patient's identification card.
- Contact the insurance carrier to determine exactly which services the patient is eligible to receive.
- Record this information on both the patient's medical record and a Verification of Benefits form.
- Provide the patient with a document listing the requirements and restrictions of their plan, and have them read and sign it.
- Collect the appropriate amount for a deductible or copayment.

Types of Health Insurance

Individual Policies: Individuals with this type of health insurance are usually ineligible to receive benefits from a government plan. This type of coverage is characterized by high premiums and a limited amount of benefits.

Group Policies: This form of insurance provides coverage for employees under a single contract. This type of coverage is characterized by greater benefits, and low premiums.

Government Plans This form of insurance is available to a large group of people who meet specific eligibility criteria. TRICARE, Medicaid, Medicare and Worker's Compensation are examples of government plans.

Mail Classifications

Express Mail This type of mail is available every day of the year, including holidays, for items up to 70 lbs in weight and 108 inches in height

First-Class Mail This type of mail includes letters, postal cards, postcards, and business reply mail

Priority Mail First-class mail that weighs more than 13 ounces

Certified Mail This type of mailing gives the sender the option to receive proof of delivery.

Bulk Mailing A form of mailing large volumes of information which is presorted by zip code.

Insurance Terms

Assignment of Benefits: An arrangement by which a patient requests that their health benefit payments be made directly to a physician

Benefit: The amount payable by the carrier toward the cost of services for which the patient is eligible for

Deductible: The amount an individual must pay for health care expenses before insurance (or a self-insured company) covers the costs. Often, insurance plans are based on yearly deductible amounts.

Copayment: The portion of a service fee that the patient must pay

Policy: A document that describes the insurance coverage for an individual or property

Premium: The amount the patient pays for an insurance contract

Usual, Customary and Reasonable (UCR) or Covered Expenses: An amount customarily charged for or covered for similar services and supplies which are medically necessary, recommended by a doctor, or required for treatment.

Waiting Period: A period of time when you are not covered by insurance for a particular problem.

Medical Records Management

Creating a Medical Record

The Medical Administrative Assistant should take the following steps to establish a patient's medical record:

- Determine the patient's status in the office (New or Established)
- Obtain the required general information
- Enter the information into the patient history form
- Review the form for accuracy
- Enter the patient's name into the computerized ledger
- Assemble the appropriate forms, prepare the folder and file as necessary

Filing

Indexing

- The Medical Administrative should use the following indexing rules:

1. Last Name, First Name, Middle Name/Initial

2. The hyphenated portion of a name is used as one unit Ex: Anna Smith-Meyer is filed as Smithmeyer, Anna

3. Apostrophes are not used in filing

4. Titles, and terms of seniority are only used to distinguish from an identical name

5. When indexing a company, articles such as "The" and "A" are not used Ex: The Mandarin Office is filed as: Mandarin Office

Alphabetical Filing

- Folders are arranged in the same sequence of the alphabet
- The medical assistant must ensure that the filing cabinet has enough space for proper distribution of the files amongst each letter of the alphabet

Numerical Filing

- An alphabetic cross-reference is used to categorize materials with digits
- Patients are assigned in a consecutive number
- Records are filed backwards in groups
- Ex: Terminal digit filing

Components of the Medical Record

Personal and Medical History

Created using information gathered from the patient. Usually includes information such as past illnesses, surgical operations, and the patient's daily health habits.

Patient's Family History

This information is just as important as the patient's personal and medical history. Includes information regarding the health of members of the patient's family, and a record of the causes of death.

Patient's Social History

Includes information regarding the patient's lifestyle. Ex: Smoking and Drinking Habits

Patient's Chief Complaint

A statement of the patient's symptoms.

Diagnosis A decision made based on the information regarding the patient's history and the results of the doctor's examination

Problem Oriented Medical Record

SOAP Approach A format for progress notes based on the letters of the word:

S: Subjective Impressions

O: Objective clinical evidence

A: Assessment or Diagnosis

P: Plans for further studies, treatment, or management

Subject Filing

☐ Either an alphabetic or alphanumeric code is assigned to general correspondence

Tickler File

☐ A collection of date labeled file folders used as a reminder for time sensitive matters or other important information

☐ Used as a follow up method

☐ Should be checked each day

Medical Terminology

Word Analysis

Healthcare terminology is broken down into word roots, prefixes, suffixes and combining vowels and forms. Word roots, or base words, are the foundation of the healthcare term. A suffix is a word ending, a prefix is a word beginning, and a combining vowel, (usually o), links the root to the suffix or to another root. The combining form is word root plus the appropriate combining vowel.

For example: oste /o/ athr/itis

Combining Forms and Their Meanings

Some combining forms and their meanings:

Arthr/o   joint

Bi/o   life

Cardi/o   heart

Carcin/o   cancerous, cancer

Cephal/o   head

Cerebr/o   cerebrum (largest part of the brain)

Cyt/o   cell

Dent/I   teeth

Derm/o   skin

Electr/o   electrical activity

Enter/o   intestines

Fet/o   fetus

Gastr/o   stomach

Hepat/o   liver

Iatr/o   treatment, physician

Leuk/o   white blood cells

Nephr/o   kidney

Oste/o   bone

Path/o   disease

Ren/o   kidney

Rhin/o   nose

Sarc/o   flesh

Thromb/o   clotting

Ur/o   urinary tract

Some suffixes and their meanings:

-al   pertaining to

-algia   pain

-dynia   pain

-ectomy   excision, removal

-emia   condition

-genic   produced by, pertaining to producing

-globin   protein

-itis   inflammation

-oma   tumor, mass swelling

-osis   condition, usually abnormal

-pathy   disease condition

-sis   state of; condition

Some Prefixes and their meanings:

Ante-   before, in front of

Anti -   against

Brady-   slow

Dia -   through, complete

End, endo   within

Epi -   above, upon

Hyper-   excessive, above more than normal

Hypo -   deficient, below, under less than normal

Peri -   surrounding, around

Pre-   before

Sub-   under, below

Suffixes used to describe therapeutic interventions

-ectomy   excision

-graphy   process of recording

-metry   process of measurement

-scopy   a visual examination

-stomy   a new opening

-tomy   incision

-tripsy   process of crushing

Suffixes used to describe instruments

-graph   an instrument/machine to record

-meter   an instrument to measure

-scope   an instrument to visually or aurally examine

-tome   an instrument to cut

-tripter   an instrument to crush

-trite   an instrument to crush

Body Structure and Directional Terminology

Body Structure Terminology

The various body systems, organs, tissues, and positional and directional terms will be addressed.

Organs

Organs are comprised of several types of tissue. The stomach is made up of muscle tissue, nerve tissue, and epithelial tissue. The medical term for internal organs is viscera. Systems are groups of organs working together to perform complex functions.

Body Systems	Functions	Organs
Musculoskeletal	support, movement, protection	muscles, bones, joints, bone marrow
Integumentary	protection	skin, hair, nails
Gastrointestinal	nutrition	stomach, intestines
Urinary	elimination of nitrogenous waste	kidneys, bladder, ureters, urethra
Reproductive	reproduction	ovaries, testes
Blood/Lymphatic	transportation	blood cells
Immune	protection	
Cardiovascular	transportation	lymph glands, heart, vessels
Respiratory	delivers O2 to cells, lungs, removes CO2	bronchi, trachea
Nervous/Behavioral	receive/process information	brain, nerves, mind
Endocrine	effects changes through pancreas, thyroid	chemical messengers

Body Cavities

The body is divided into five cavities. Two of these cavities are in the back of the body and are called dorsal cavities. The positional term is posterior. The other three cavities are in the front of the body and are called ventral cavities. The positional term is called anterior. The cranial cavity and the spinal cavity are the two dorsal cavities. The ventral cavities are the thoracic cavity which is divided into two smaller cavities; the pleural and the mediastinum. The pleural cavity is the space surrounding each lung, and the mediastinum contains the heart, aorta, trachea, etc. The diaphragm, a muscle, separates the thoracic cavity from the abdominal cavity. The abdominal cavity contains the stomach, the small and large intestines, spleen, pancreas, liver and gallbladder. The pelvic cavity contains the rectum, urinary bladder, urethra and ureters; uterus and vagina in the female. Due to the fact that there is nothing that separates the abdominal cavity and the pelvic cavity, they are often referred to as the abdominopelvic cavity.

Planes of the Body

Dividing the body into planes or flat surfaces is an additional way to describe the body. These descriptions listed below are useful when doing magnetic imaging, CT scans, and other imaging techniques.

Sagittal planes are vertical planes that separate the sides from each other.

Midsagittal plane separates the body into right and left halves.

The frontal plane divides the body into front and back portions. The transverse plane divides the body horizontally into an upper and lower part.

Positional and Directional Terms

Anterior (ventral) – front surface of the body

Posterior (dorsal) – back side of the body

Deep – away from the surface

Proximal –near the point of attachment to the trunk or near the beginning of a structure.

Distal – far from the point of attachment to the trunk or far from the beginning of a structure.

Inferior – below another structure

Superior – above another structure Medial – pertaining to the middle or nearer the medial plane of the body

Lateral – pertaining to the side

Supine – lying on the back

Prone – lying on the belly

Musculoskeletal System

The musculoskeletal system includes the bones, muscles, and joints. The bones are connected to one another by fibrous bands of tissue called ligaments. Muscles are attached to the bone by tendons. The fibrous covering of the muscles is called the fascia and the articular cartilage covers the end of many bones and serves as a protective function. The musculoskeletal system acts as a framework for the organs, protects many of those organs, and also provides the organism the ability to move.

Bones

Bones are complete organs made up of connective tissue called osseous. The inner core of bones is comprised of hematopoietic tissue. This is where the red bone marrow manufactures blood cells. Other parts of the bone are storage areas for minerals necessary for growth. Examples of these minerals are calcium and phosphorous.

Types of bones

Bones are categorized as belonging to either the axial skeleton or the appendicular skeleton. The axial skeleton consists of the skull, rib cage, and spine. The appendicular skeleton is made up of the shoulder, collar, pelvic and arms and legs.

Bones come in a variety of shapes and sizes. The following is a description of shapes of human bones and where they are located.

Long bones are typically very strong, are broad at the ends and have large surfaces for muscle attachment. The humerus and the femur are large bones. Short bones are small with irregular shapes. They are found in the wrist and ankle. Flat bones are found covering soft body parts. These are the shoulder blades, ribs, and pelvic bones. Sesamoid bones are small, rounded bones that resemble a sesame seed. They are found near joints and increase the efficiency of muscles near a joint. An example of sesamoid bone is the knee cap.

The Axial Skeleton – Skull, Spine, Rib Cage

The skull is made up of two parts, the cranium and the facial bones. The cranium includes the following bones: Frontal Bone – forms the anterior part of the skull and the forehead Parietal Bones – forms the sides of the cranium Occipital Bone – forms the back of the skull. There is a large hole at the ventral surface in this bone, called the foramen magnum, which allows the brain communication with the spinal cord. Temporal Bone – forms the two lower sides of the cranium. Ethmoid Bone – forms the roof of the nasal cavity. Sphenoid Bones – anterior to the temporal bones.

Facial Bones

Zygoma – Cheekbone Lacrimal bones – paired bones at the corner of each eye that cradle the tear ducts. Maxilla – upper jaw bone Mandible – lower jaw bone Vomer – bone that forms posterior/inferior part of the nasal septal wall between the nostrils. Palatine bones – make up part of the roof of the mouth Inferior nasal conchae – make up part of the interior of the nose.

Spinal/Vertebral Column

The spinal /vertebral column is divided into five regions from the neck to the tailbone. There are 26 bones in the spine and they are referred to as the vertebrae. The following list explains the bones of the spine Cervical Neck Bones Thoracic Upper back Lumbar Lower back Sacral Sacrum Coccygeal Coccyx (tailbone)

Rib Cage

There are 12 pairs of ribs. The first 7 pairs join the sternum anteriorly through cartilaginous attachments called costal cartilages. The true ribs, numbers 1-7, attach directly to the sternum in the front of the body. False ribs, numbers 8-10, are attached to the sternum by cartilage. Ribs 11 and 12 are floating ribs, because they are not attached at all.

The Appendicular Skeleton

The upper appendicular skeleton includes the shoulder girdle which is made up of the scapula, clavicle and upper extremities. The scapula, or shoulder blades are flat bones that help support the arms. The clavicle, or collarbone, is curved horizontal bones that attach to the upper sternum at one end. These bones help stabilize the shoulder. The upper extremities consist of the following: The humerus which is the upper arm bone. The ulna is the lower medial arm bone. The radius is the lateral lower arm bone (in line with the thumb). The carpals are wrist bones. There are 2 rows of four bones in the wrist. The metacarpals are the five radiating bones in the fingers. These are the bones in the palm of the hand. The phalanges (phalanx.s) are the finger bones. Each finger has three phalanges, except for the thumb. The three phalanges are the proximal, middle and a distal phalanx. The thumb has a proximal and distal.

Lower Appendicular

The lower half of the appendicular skeleton can be divided into the pelvis and the lower extremities. Pelvis: superior and widest bone Ischium: lower portion of the pelvic bone Pubic bone: the lower anterior part of the bone

Lower Extremities

Femur: thighbone Patella: kneecap Tibia: shin Fibula: smaller, lateral leg bone Malleolus: ankle Tarsal: hind foot bone Metatarsal: midfoot bone Phalanx: toe bones, 14 in all (2 in the great toe, 3 in each of the other toes)

Joints

The joints are the parts of the body where two or more bones of the skeleton join. Different joints have different ROM (range of motion), ranging from no movement at all to full range of movement.

No ROM – most synarthroses are immovable joints held together by fibrous tissue.

Limited ROM- amphiathroses are joints joined together by cartilage that is slightly moveable, such as the vertebrae of the spine or the pubic bone.

Full ROM – diathroses are joints that have free movement. Ball-and-socket joints (hip) and hinge joints (knees) are common diathroses joints. (synovial joints)

Synovial joints, free moving joints, are surrounded by joint capsules. Many of the synovial joints have bursae, which are sacs of fluid that are located between the bones of the joint and the tendons that hold the muscles in place.

Muscles

Muscle is tissue composed of cells. Muscles have the ability to contract and relax. The muscles in the human body have three different functions: 1. to allow the skeleton to move, 2. responsible for movement of organs, and 3. to pump blood to the circulatory system. Muscles are attached to bones by strong, fibrous bands of connective tissue called tendons.

Muscle Actions

Action	Description
Extension	to increase the angle of a joint
Flexion	to decrease the angle of a joint
Abduction	movement away from the midline
Adduction	movement towards the midline
Supination	turning the palm or foot upward
Pronation	turning the palm or foot downward
Dorsiflexion	raising the foot, pulling the toes toward the shin

Plantar flexion — lowering the foot, pointing the toes away from the shin

Eversion — turning outward

Inversion — turning inward

Protraction — moving a part of the body forward

Retraction — moving a part of the body backward

Rotation — revolving a bone around its axis

Fractures

A fracture is a broken bone. Most fractures occur as a result of trauma, however some diseases like cancer or osteoporosis can also cause spontaneous fractures. Fractures can be classified as simple or compound. Simple fractures do not rupture the skin, as compound fractures split open the skin allowing for an infection to occur.

Types of Fractures

Comminuted – the bone is crushed and or shattered.

Compression – the fractured area of bone collapses on itself.

Colles – the break of the distal end of the radius at the epiphysis often occurs when the patient has attempted to break his or her fall.

Complicated – the bone is broken and pierces an internal organ

Impacted – the bone is broken and the ends are driven into each other.

Hairline – A minor fracture appears as a thin line on x-ray and may not extend completely through the bone.

Greenstick – the bone is partially bent and partially broken; this is a common fracture in children because their bones are still soft.

Pathologic – any fracture occurring spontaneously as a result of disease.

Salter-Harris – a fracture of the epiphyseal plate in children.

Sprains, strains and dislocation/subluxation: A sprain is a traumatic injury to a joint involving the soft tissue. The soft tissue includes, the muscles, ligaments, and tendons. A strain is a lesser injury, usually this is a result of overuse or overstretching. Dislocation is when a bone is completely out of place and subluxation is partially out of joint.

The Integumentary System

The skin and its accessory organs make up the integumentary system. Integument means covering. The skin covers over an area of 22 square feet (an average adult). It is a complex system of specialized tissues containing glands, nerves and blood vessels. The main function of the skin is to protect the deeper tissues from excessive loss of minerals, heat, and water. It also provides protects the body from diseases by providing a barrier. The skin is the largest organ of the body and accomplishes its diverse functions with assistance from the hair, nails, and glands. The sebaceous(oil) glands and the suddoriferous (sweat) glands produce secretions that allow the body to be moisturized or cooled. Nerve fibers help the body adjust to the environment by sensory messages relayed to the brain and spinal cord. Other tissues in the skin maintain body temperature. Nerve fibers also help blood vessels to dilate and sweat gland to produce sweat.

There are three layers to the skin: the epidermis, the dermis, and the subcutaneous layer. The epidermis is a thin, cellular membrane layer that contains keratin. The dermis is a dense, fibrous, connective tissue that contains collagen. The subcutaneous layer is a thicker and fatter tissue.

Hair, Nails and Glands

Hair fibers are composed of tightly fused meshwork of cells filled with hard protein called keratin. The hair has its roots in the dermis and together with their coverings, is called hair follicles. The main function of the hair is to assist in the regulation of body temperature. It holds heat in when the body is cold by standing on end and holding a layer of air as insulation.

Nails cover and protect the dorsal surfaces of the distal bones of the fingers and toes. The part that is visible is the nail body, the nail root is under skin at the base of the nail and the nail bed is the vascular tissue under the nail that appears pink when the blood is oxygenated or blue/purple when it is oxygen deficient. The moon like white area at the base of the nail is called the lunula. There is also the cuticle at the lower part of the nail and this is sometimes referred to as the eponychium.

Sebaceous glands are located in the dermal layer of the skin over the entire body, except for the palms of the hands and soles of the feet. The sebaceous glands secrete an oily substance called sebum. Sebum contains lipids that help lubricate the skin and minimize water loss. It is the overproduction of sebum during puberty that contributes to acne in some people.

Sweat glands are tiny, coiled gland found on almost all body surfaces. They are most numerous in the palms and soles of the feet. Coiled sweat glands originate in the dermis and straighten out to extend up through the epidermis. The tiny opening on the surface is a pore. There are two types of sweat glands: eccrine sweat glands are the most common and the apocrine sweat glands that secrete an odorless sweat.

Integumentary Vocabulary

Albino- deficient in pigment (melanin)

Collagen- structural protein found in the skin and connective tissue

Melanin- major skin pigment

Lipocyte- a fat cell

Macule- discolored, flat lesion (freckles, tattoo marks)

Polyp benign growth extending from the surface of the mucous membrane

Fissure- groove or crack like sore

Nodule- solid, round or oval elevated lesion more than 1 cm in diameter

Ulcer- open sore on the skin or mucous membranes

Vesicle- small collection of clear fluid; blister

Wheal- smooth, slightly elevated, edematous(swollen) area that is redder or paler than the surrounding skin.

Alopecia- absence of hair from areas where it normally grows

Gangrene- death of tissue associated with loss of blood supply

Impetigo- bacterial inflammatory skin disease characterized by lesion, pustules and vesicles.

Practice Test:

1. Which of the following is NOT a "hard copy"

a. A record printed on paper

b. A faxed copy of a document

c. An unprinted file saved to a computer

d. A typewritten report received in the mail

2. Arbitration means:

a. Both parties agree to use a mediator to settle any disputes regarding medical care

b. A patient cannot bring suit against a physician for malpractice

c. Physicians have to be held harmless in case of medical mishaps

d. The same as the Good Samaritan act

3. Certified mail provides the sender with:

a. Insurance protection

b. An inexpensive way to send valuables

c. Quick delivery

d. Proof of delivery

4 Which reference book is used to check for the correct spelling of drugs:

a. Standard dictionary

b. Physician's desk reference

c. Medical dictionary

d. Current procedural terminology

5 Which of the following is the correct filing order for Dave Jonson, Nancy Johnenson, Susan Johnson and Johnny Johanson.

a. Nancy Johenson, Susan Johnson, Dave Jonson, Johnny Johanson

b. Dave Jonson, Johnny Johanson, Nancy Johenson, Susan Johnson

c. Johnny Johanson, Nancy Johnenson, Susan Johnson, Dave Jonson

d. Johnny Johanson, Dave Jonson, Nancy Johenson, Susan Johnson

6 In the chart number "12345.10", the numbers following the "." (decimal) are:

a. Filed last

b. Terminal digits

c. Alphabetical indicators

d. For insurance companies only

7 The total of all amounts due to the physician, from all patients, for services rendered or procedures performed is called the:

a. Assets

b. Liabilities

c. Accounts payable

d. Accounts receivable

8 When asked about a patient's condition by the family, the medical administrative assistant should:

a. Put it in writing rather than speak directly

b. Tell them what they want to know

c. Obtain permission from the patient

d. Tell the family it is not their concern

9 A patient with a hyphenated last name should have a rolodex card or other notation made of both last names. This procedure is called:

a. Correlation

b. Re-routing

c. Continuance

d. Cross-referencing

10 If a physician decides to end the professional relationship with a patient, what must the physician do to help avoid being sued for abandonment?

a. Call the patient personally and explain that the physician is withdrawing from the case.

b. The physician immediately sends the record to another physician believed to be competent to handle the case.

c. Thoroughly document, in writing – to the patient – the reason for withdrawing from the case and stipulate a specified number of days for the patient to seek a new physician

d. Return any money collected

11. The symptoms a patient is currently seen for are called:

a. The prognosis

b. The diagnosis

c. The patient record

d. The chief complaint

12. Giving the patient adequate information concerning the method, risk and consequences prior to a procedure is called:

a. Confidentiality

b. Tort

c. The right to know

d. Informed consent

13 The letters S, O, A, and P in SOAP format for progress notes, stand for

a. Source, order, assessment, prognosis

b. Start, objective, align, plan

c. Subjective, objective, assessment, plan

d. Selection, objection, appeal, prognosis

14. A medical administrative assistant's duties include all of the following except:

a. Patient reception

b. Filing Medical Records

c. Performing EKGs

d. Setting up Appointments

15. In order to verify insurance coverage you should:

a. Ask the patient if their coverage is effective

b. Copy their card for the file

c. Call the insurance carrier for verification of current coverage

d. Check the effective date on their insurance card

16. Which of the following would be filed THIRD?

a. 134356

b. 143679

c. 127890

d. 109456

17. The "Inside Address" in a typewritten letter would include:

a. The name and address of the person sending the letter

b. The name and address of the person receiving the letter

c. The salutation

d. The body of the letter

18 A form of mailing large volumes of information, where you pre-sort your mail by zip code, then take it to the post-office for delivery is called:

a. Certified mail

b. UPS

c. Bulk mailing

d. Zip coding

19. The "amount" that an insurance company may say is "not allowed" and not the responsibility of the patient, for a contracted physician, would become "what" on the patient's account?

a. A charge

b. An adjustment

c. A payment

d. A deductible

20 Sue Tomas has group insurance. She was charged $75 for an office visit and $25.00 for a complete blood count, totaling $100.00. Her group insurance paid 80% of the charges. How much did they pay?

a. $ 100.00

b. $ 20.00

c. $ 80.00

d. $ 75.00

ANSWER KEY
1 C
2 A
3 D
4 B
5 C
6 B
7 D
8 C
9 D
10 C
11 D
12 D
13 C
14 C
15 C
16 A
17 B
18 C
19 B
20 C

SECTION TWO

Infection Control

The chain of infection requires a continuous link among three elements:

Source --------------------------- Transmission --------------------- Susceptible host

        Portal   Portal

          of   of

         Exit   Entry

The source refers to the location of the pathogenic organism. Transmission is the method by which the microorganism is transferred to the susceptible host, which could be the patient, or for that matter, any person.

The microorganism must have a means to get out of the source (portal of exit) and a means to get inside the susceptible host (portal of entry) to complete the chain of infection. The goal of biologic safety is to prevent this completion of the chain. Specific safety practices are directed toward each component with the goal of breaking it.

An infection contracted by the patient during hospitalization is called "Nosocomial Infection."

Health care providers, not following instituted control practices, cause most of these infections.

Hand contact is the most common method of transmission, which is why hand washing is the most important means of prevention.

Isolation Precautions

For many years, the CDC recommended universal precautions, which is a method of infection control that assumed that all human blood and body fluids were potentially infectious. The CDC issued a revised guidelines consisting of two tiers or levels of precautions: Standard Precautions and Transmission-Based Precautions.

Standard Precautions

This is an infection control method designed to prevent direct contact with blood and other body fluids and tissues by using barrier protection and work control practices.

Under the standard precautions, all patients are presumed to be infective for blood-borne pathogens. Infection control practices to be used with all patients. These replace universal precautions and body substance isolation. They are used when there is a possibility of contact with any of the following:

Blood

All body fluids, secretions, and excretions (except sweat), regardless of whether or not they contain visible blood

Nonintact skin

Mucous membranes designed to reduce the risk of transmission of microorganisms from both Recognized and unrecognized sources of infections.

The standard precautions are:

Wear gloves when collecting and handling blood, body fluids, or tissue specimen. Wear face shields when there is a danger for splashing on mucous membranes. Dispose of all needles and sharp objects in puncture-proof containers without recapping.

Transmission- Based Precautions the second tier of precautions and are to be used when the patient is known or suspected of being infected with contagious disease. They are to be used in addition to standard precautions.

All types of isolation are condensed into three categories:

Contact precautions: are designed to reduce the risk of transmission of microorganisms by direct or indirect contact. Direct-contact transmission involves skin-to-skin contact and physical transfer of microorganisms to a susceptible host from an infected or colonized person. Indirect-contact transmission involves contact with a contaminated intermediate object in the patient's environment.

Airborne precautions: are designed to reduce the risk of airborne transmission of infectious agents. Microorganisms carried in this manner can be dispersed widely by air currents and may become inhaled by or deposited on a susceptible host within the same room or over a longer distance from the source patient. Special air handling and ventilation are required to prevent airborne transmission.

Droplet precautions: are designed to reduce the risk of droplet transmission of infectious agents. Droplet transmission involves contact with the conjunctivae or the mucous membranes of the nose or mouth of a susceptible person with large particle droplets generated from the source person primarily during coughing, sneezing, or talking. Because droplets generally travel only short distances, usually three feet or less, and do not remain suspended in the air, special air handling and ventilation are not required.

Hepatitis and Acquired Immunodeficiency Syndrome (AIDS)

Hepatitis and acquired immunodeficiency syndrome (AIDS) represent constant threats to the health and safety of laboratory personnel. Both of these potentially deadly diseases are transmitted as a result of exposure to blood and body fluids from an infected individual. The infectious process is similar for both of these diseases.

Hepatitis A

Type A virus causes Hepatitis A (HAV) previously called "infectious hepatitis". It is usually spread by the fecal-oral route as a result of improper personal hygiene methods or consumption of contaminated foods, such as shellfish. It is a very common form of viral hepatitis; indeed, approximately 143,000 cases were reported in the United States in 1994.

Hepatitis B

Hepatitis B (HBV), previously referred to as serum hepatitis, is caused by type B virus and is acquired parenterally, through contact with blood (transfusions, hypodermic needles, dental and surgical instruments) and body fluids (tears, saliva, and semen). People who collect and process blood are considered to be at high risk for contracting HBV. Although most infected individuals recover, 10% of the population with HBV become chronic carriers.

Hepatitis B Immunization

OSHA standards require physicians to offer the hepatitis B vaccination series, free of charge, to all medical office personnel who may have occupational exposure. It is a three-dose series that is believed to give immunity to the virus. The immunization must be offered within the first 10 days of employment in an occupational risk area. Laboratory personnel who do not want to be vaccinated must sign a waiver form documenting refusal, which is to be filled in the employee's OSHA record.

AIDS

AIDS is not a disease that can be casually contracted. Routine encounters with patients in the laboratory are not sources of HIV transmission. Comparing all the sexually transmitted diseases that are known to us, HIV is the most difficult to contract. Although the chances of contracting HIV are low, the serious nature of the infection makes it imperative that the laboratory assistant use precautionary procedures. AIDS is caused by a retrovirus known as HIV.

Because many HIV carriers are asymptomatic and may not be aware that they have the virus, procedures to minimize the risk of exposure to blood and body fluids should be taken with all patients at all times. The current guidelines for diagnosing AIDS are based on the following criteria: (1) the presence of AIDS-related disorders, and (2) the T-cell count of an HIV-infected individual. The normal range for the T-cell count is 800 to 1600/cm of blood. The diagnosis of AIDS is applied to individuals with a T-cell count of 200/cm or less.

Needle Stick Prevention Act

OSHA has put into force the Occupational Exposure to Bloodborne pathogen (BBP) Standard when it was concluded that healthcare employees face a serious health risk as a result of occupational exposure to blood and other body fluids and tissues. The standards outline necessary engineering and work practice controls that OSHA believes will help minimize or eliminate exposure to employees. The standard was revised in 2001 to conform to the Needlestick Safety and Prevention Act passed in November 2000. The act directed OSHA to revise the BBP standard in four key areas:

- Revision and updating of the exposure control plan.
- Solicitation of employee input in selecting engineering and work practice controls.

☐ Modification of definitions relating to engineering controls (i.e., sharps disposal containers, self-sheathing needles, needleless systems.

☐ New record keeping requirements.

The employer must establish and maintain a sharps injury log for percutaneous injury from contaminated sharps and it must be done in such a manner to protect the confidentiality of the injured employee.

The sharps injury log must contain, at a minimum:

a. The type and brand of device involved in the incident.

b. The department or work area where the exposure incident occurred.

c. An explanation of how the incident occurred.

** See Appendix B for further clarification.

Latex Sensitivity

Latex sensitivity is an emerging and important problem in the health care field. Following the development of Universal Precaution Standards (OSHA, 1980), the use of natural rubber latex gloves for infection control skyrocketed. Within the last decade, however, the incidence of latex sensitivity has grown. It is an issue that every health care worker must be concerned about.

Individuals with a known sensitivity to latex should wear a medical alert bracelet.

APPENDIX A: PATIENTS BILL OF RIGHTS

As a patient in XXX Hospital you have the right, consistent with law, to:

1. Receive treatment without discrimination as to race, color, religion, gender, national origin, disability, or source of payment.

2. Receive considerate and respectful care in a clean and safe environment free of unnecessary restraints.

3. Receive emergency care if you need it.

4. Be informed of the name and position of the doctor who will be in charge of your care in the hospital.

5. Know the names, positions and functions of any hospital staff involved in your care.

6. Receive complete information about your diagnosis, treatment and prognosis.

7. Receive all the information that you need to give informed consent for any proposed procedure or treatment. This information shall include the possible risks and benefits of the procedure or treatment.

8. Receive all the information you need to give informed consent for an order not to resuscitate. You also have the right to designate an individual to give this consent for you if you are too ill to do so. If you would like additional information, please ask

9. Refuse treatment, examination, or observation, if retired or a family member, and be told what effect this may have on your health.

10. Refuse to take part in research. In deciding whether or not to participate, you have the right to a full explanation.

11. Privacy while in the hospital and confidentiality of all information and records regarding your care.

12. Participate in all decisions about your treatment and discharge from the hospital.

13. Review your medical record without charge. Obtain a copy of your medical record for which the hospital can charge a reasonable fee. You cannot be denied a copy solely because you cannot afford to pay.

14. Receive a bill and explanation of all charges.

15. Complain without fears of reprisals about the care and services you are receiving and to have the hospital respond to you; and if requested, a written response. If you are not satisfied with the hospital's response, you can complain to the Patient Representative Office located in the hospital.

16. Receive information about pain and pain relief measures, be involved in pain management plan, and receive a quick response to reports of pain.

17. Receive healthcare in an environment that is dedicated to avoiding patient harm and improving patient safety.

18. The right to request information about advance directives regarding your decisions about medical care.

19. Make known your wishes in regard to anatomical gifts. Your may document your wishes in your health care proxy or on

a donor card, available from the hospital.

20. Understand and use these rights. If for any reason you do not understand or you need help, the hospital will attempt to provide assistance, including an interpreter.

Patient Responsibilities

Provision of Information: You have the responsibility to provide, to the best of your knowledge, accurate and complete information about present complaints, past illness, hospitalizations, medications, and other matters relating to your health. You have the responsibility to report unexpected changes in your condition to the responsible practitioner. You are responsible for making it known whether you clearly comprehend a contemplated course of action and what is expected of you.

Compliance with Instructions: You are responsible for following the treatment plan recommended by the practitioner primarily responsible for your care. This may include following the instructions of nurses and allied health personnel as they carry out the coordinated plan of care and implement the responsible practitioner's orders, and as they enforce the applicable hospital rules and regulations. You are responsible for keeping appointments and, when you are unable to do so for any reason, for notifying the responsible practitioner or the hospital.

Refusal of Treatment: You are responsible for your actions if you refuse treatment or do not follow the practitioner's instructions.

Hospital Rules and Regulations: You are responsible for following hospital rules and regulation affecting patient care and conduct.

Respect and Consideration: You are responsible for being considerate of the rights of other patients and hospital personnel and for assisting in the control of noise, smoking and the number of visitors. You are responsible for being respectful of the property of other persons and the hospital.

Patient Representative

The Patient Representative's primary assignment is to assist you in exercising your rights as a patient. He/she is also available to act as your advocate and to provide a specific channel through which you can seek solutions to problems, concerns and unmet needs. You may call the Patient Representative at (000)000-0000.

The Patient Bill of Rights for Pain Management

You have the right to:

-Information about pain and pain relief

-A caring staff who believe your reports of pain

-A care staff with concern about your pain

-A quick response when you report your pain

-You have the responsibility to:

-Ask for pain relief when your pain first starts

-Help those caring for you to assess your pain

-Tell those caring for you if your pain is not relieved

-Tell those caring for you about any worries that you have about taking pain medications

-Decide if you want your family and/or significant others to aid in your relief of illness

Multiple Choice Questions

1) Which of the following is a way to prevent infection spread?
    a. Wearing gloves
    b. Proper hand washing
    c. Isolating infected body substances
    d. All of the above

2) Which of the following is true about medical asepsis?
    a. It eliminates risk of infection spread
    b. It aims at destroying pathologic organisms
    c. It is necessary to use on all patients
    d. All of the above

3) Chain of infection is defined as:
    a. Links, each of which is necessary for disease to spread
    b. The method of which an infectious agent leaves its reservoir
    c. Infectious microorganisms that can be classified into groups
    d. None of the above

4) Which of the following is not an agent of infection?
    a. Virus
    b. Fungi
    c. Host
    d. Parasite
    e. bacteria

5) Which of the following is not part of the chain of infection?
    a. Portal of exit
    b. Agents
    c. Mode of transportation

d. Mode of transmission

6) Which of the following must be interrupted in order to break the chain of infection?
    a. Portal of exit
    b. Agents
    c. Mode of transmission
    d. Any of the above

7) Which of the following is an example of droplet transmission?
    a. Contracting an illness when a co-worker sneezes
    b. Contracting an illness from contact with blood
    c. Contracting an illness by touching a surface
    d. Contracting an illness from a mosquito bite

8) Which of the following is an example of contact transmission?
    a. Contracting an illness when a co-worker sneezes
    b. Contracting an illness from contact with blood
    c. Contracting an illness from a patient with lice
    d. Contracting an illness from a mosquito bite

9) Which of the following on a human body could be a portal of exit?
    a. The liver
    b. The spleen
    c. The mouth
    d. The stomach

10) Which of the following on the human body could be a portal of entry?
    a. Smooth, unbroken skin
    b. Veins
    c. Arterioles
    d. Mucous membranes

11) Which of the following allows the infectious agent into a susceptible host?
    a. Portal of entry

b. Portal of exit

c. Agents

d. Mode of transmission

12) Which of the following patients best represents a susceptible host?

   a. A teenager coming in for a sports physical

   b. A child coming in for a school physical

   c. A baby coming in for a well child checkup

   d. A premature infant

13) Which of the following is an example of medical asepsis?

   a. Hand washing

   b. Disinfecting a room

   c. Using gloves

   d. All of the above

14) Which of the following is an example of barrier protection?

   a. Hand washing

   b. Disinfecting a room

   c. Wearing gloves

   d. All of the above

15) Which of the following is an example of barrier protection?

   a. Goggles

   b. Face shields

   c. Gloves

   d. All of the above

16) Which of the following is meant to prevent direct contact with blood and body fluids?

   a. Transmission-based precautions

   b. Standard precautions

   d. Basic precautions

   e. None of the above

17) Which of the following is not a standard precaution?
    a. Wearing gloves
    b. Recapping a sharp
    c. Wearing a mask
    d. All are standard precautions
    e. None are standard precautions

18) Which patient would you use transmission-based precautions for?
    a. A patient coming in for a physical
    b. A patient with heart problems
    c. A patient with tuberculosis
    d. A patient with a broken arm
    e. All of the above

19) Which of the following are types of transmission-based precautions?
    a. Contact precautions
    b. Airborne precautions
    c. Droplet precautions
    d. All of the above

20) Which of the following would prevent microorganisms from being dispersed to susceptible host by air currents?
    a. Contact precautions
    b. Airborne precautions
    c. Droplet precautions
    d. All of the above
    e. B and C only

21) Which of the following would prevent contamination from large particle droplets?
    a. Contact precautions
    b. Airborne precautions
    c. Droplet precautions
    d. All of the above

e. B and C only

22) Which of the following would prevent contamination from physical transfer?

　a. Contact precautions

　b. Airborne precautions

　c. Droplet precautions

　d. All of the above

　e. B and C only

23) Which department is responsible for identifying and minimizing workplace hazards?

　a. OSHA

　b. NSA

　c. ASHO

　d. NASA

　e. Security

24) What types hazards are identified workplace hazards?

　a. Biologic

　b. Chemical

　c. Electrical

　d. All of the above

25) Which of the following is an example of a physical workplace hazard?

　a. Bunsen burners

　b. Cleaning agents

　c. Wet floors

　d. Lancets

　e. Fungi

26) Which of the following is an example of a biological workplace hazard?

　a. Glass on the floor

　b. Exposed electrical wires

　c. Heavy lifting

　d. Wet floors

e. Mold on the walls

27) A coworker has slipped on the floor and broken an arm. You should:
   a. Apply pressure
   b. Elevate the arm
   c. Set the arm
   d. Get help

28) Which of the following is not a symptom of shock?
   a. Rapid, weak pulse
   b. Deep breathing
   c. Expressionless, staring eyes
   d. Pale, clammy skin

29) When a person is in shock you should not do which of the following?
   a. Call for assistance
   b. Keep the victim warm
   c. Have the patient stand up
   d. Maintain an open airway
   e. All of the above are good remedies for shock

30) Which of the following is essential for maintaining good legal practices?
   a. Practicing confidentiality
   b. Giving information to all family members
   c. Doing whatever it takes to get the blood drawn
   d. All of the above are good legal practices

31) When a patient refuses to sign a particular consent, the CMAA should:
   a. Deny her from seeing the doctor
   b. Listen to her concerns about the document
   c. Explain why the consent is important
   d. All of the above
   e. B & C

32) It is part of the patient's rights to refuse treatment.

   a. True

   b. False

33) Which of the following is not an element of negligence?

   a. Duty of care

   b. Derelict of duty

   c. Direct cause of injury

   d. Damage

   e. Draining of assets

34) Which of the following protects people rendering aid at the scene of an accident or injury?

   a. Healthcare provider protection act

   b. First responder laws

   c. Good Samaritan laws

   d. None of the above

35) Which of the following is not a common cause for tort in the healthcare field?

   a. Invasion of privacy

   b. Rendering aid

   c. Battery

   d. Defamation of character

Answers

1) D
2) D
3) A
4) C
5) C
6) D
7) A
8) C
9) C
10) D
11) A
12) D
13) D
14) C
15) D
16) A
17) A
18) C
19) D
20) B
21) E
22) A
23) A
24) D
25) C
26) E
27) D
28) B
29) C
30) A

31) E

32) A

33) E

34) C

35) B

Note that these review questions were not derived from this study guide, but were compiled to test general knowledge in preparation for the CMAA test.

Review Questions
Test 1

1. Which of this is not a useful skill for physically active learning?
    a. Walking and talking aloud while studying
    b. Using pictures to represent materials being studied
    c. Getting anxious while studying
    d. Over-learning a topic

2. Which of this is not a method of remembering materials taught in class?
    a. Quickly reviewing materials after class
    b. Creating songs for materials learnt
    c. Teaching it to someone else
    d. Studying another material when you don't understand the one being taught

3. _____ is not a Mind map that helps consolidate complex details and organize them in a format easy to remember?
    a. Spider Map
    b. Octopus Map
    c. Chain of event Map
    d. Fish-bone Map

4. _____ is a key to critical thinking?

a. Reflection
b. Learning
c. Information
d. Knowledge

5. The way an individual perceives and processes information to learn new material is called?
   a. Perceiving
   b. Processing
   c. Learning style
   d. Critical thinking

6. The constant practice of considering all aspects of a situation when deciding what to believe or what to do is called?
   a. Professional Behavior
   b. Reflection
   c. Critical thinking
   d. LearningStyle

7. The process of considering new information and internalizing it to create new ways of examining information is called?
   a. Processing
   b. Examining
   c. Reflection
   d. Perceiving

8. How an individual internalizes new information and makes it his or her own is called?
   a. Processing
   b. Examining
   c. Reflection
   d. Perceiving

9. The actions that identify the medical assistant as a member of a healthcare profession including being dependable, performing respectful patient care, demonstrating positive attitude and using teamwork is called?

a. Healthcare behaviors

b. Professional behaviors

c. Medical Assistant actions

d. Successful medical assistant student

10. For you to learn new materials you must _____ and _____ information?

   a. Perceive and Process

   b. Investigate and Learn

   c. Access and Examine

   d. Internalize and Perceive

11. Learners perceive information in 2 ways?

   a. Active and passive

   b. Appropriate and inappropriate

   c. Learnt and Unlearnt

   d. Concrete and Abstract

12. Learners with a concrete reflective style like to?

   a. Consider a situation from many different point of view

   b. Learn lots of facts and arrange new materials in a logical and clear manner

   c. Know how techniques and ideas work

   d. Relate new materials to other areas in their life

13. Learners with an Abstract reflective style like to?

   a. Consider a situation from many different point of view

   b. Learn lots of facts and arrange new materials in a logical and clear manner

   c. Know how techniques and ideas work

   d. Relate new materials to other areas in their life

14. Learners with a concrete active style like to?

   a. Consider a situation from many different point of view

   b. Learn lots of facts and arrange new materials in a logical and clear manner

   c. Know how techniques and ideas work

d. Relate new materials to other areas in their life

15. Which of this is not a time management skill?
    a. Setting aside time to do things you enjoy
    b. Avoid working on long term goals
    c. Identify your main concern
    d. Determining your purpose

16. An enzymatically controlled transformation of an organic compound is called?
    a. Contamination
    b. Fermentation
    c. Organic
    d. All of the above

17. A type of alternative medicine that attempts to stimulate the body to recover itself is called?
    a. Naturopathy
    b. Homeopathy
    c. Osteopathic
    d. Hospice

18. Slight misalignment of the vertebrae or partial dislocation is?
    a. Sprain
    b. Strain
    c. Subluxation
    d. Sublimation

19. The use of telecommunications devices to enhance and improve the results of radiologic procedures is?
    a. Telemedicine
    b. Teleradiology
    c. Televice
    d. All of the above

20. A condition in which majority of the people in a country or a geographical area are affected is called?

a. Endemic

b. Pandemic

c. Osteopathic

d. Mysticism

21. The experience of seeming to have direct communication with God or ultimate reality is?

    a. Mystery

    b. Spirituality

    c. Holistic

    d. Mysticism

22. Which of this eradication is the greatest accomplishment of World Health Organization (WHO)?

    a. Polio

    b. Leprosy

    c. Chickenpox

    d. Smallpox

23. Which of these agencies created the ICD-9?

    a. United Nations

    b. World Health Organization

    c. U.S. Department of Health and Human Services

    d. National Institute of Health

24. _____ is the principal U.S agency for providing essential human services and protecting the health of all Americans?

    a. U.S Medical Institute

    b. World Health Organization

    c. U.S. Department of Health and Human Services (HHS)

    d. National Institute of Health

25. Which of the following is not pathogen studied at biosafety IV?

    a. Influenza virus

    b. Ebola Virus

    c. Lassa Virus

d. Hantavirus

26. _____ is the principal U.S. federal agency concerned with the health and safety of people throughout the world as his part of HHS?
   a. United Nations
   b. World Health Organization
   c. Centers for Disease Control and Prevention
   d. National Institute of Health

27. Which of this is not a type of health care facility?
   a. Hospital
   b. Ambulatory care
   c. All of the above
   d. None of the above

28. Which of this is not a type of business structure that exists in the medical practice?
   a. Sole Proprietorship
   b. Limited Proprietorship
   c. Partnership
   d. Corporation

29. _____ is defined as an artificial entity having a legal and business status that is independent of its shareholders or employees?
   a. Sole Proprietorship
   b. Limited Proprietorship
   c. Partnership
   d. Corporation

30. Which of the following is the owner potentially liable for all of the acts of his or her professional employees and staff members?
   a. Sole Proprietorship
   b. Limited Proprietorship
   c. Partnership
   d. Corporation

31. Which of this has the disadvantage where each physician is liable for the actions and conduct of the other?
    a. Sole Proprietorship
    b. Limited Proprietorship
    c. Partnership
    d. Corporation

32. When an individual holds exclusive rights and title to all aspect of the medical practice is called?
    a. Sole Proprietorship
    b. Limited Proprietorship
    c. Partnership
    d. Corporation

33. This specialist uses radioactive substances for the diagnosis and treatment of diseases?
    a. Neurological Surgeon
    b. Nuclear Medicine Specialist
    c. Anesthesiologist
    d. Urologist

34. The medical specialist concerned with the treatment of disease and disorders of the urinary tract is?
    a. Neurological Surgeon
    b. Nuclear Medicine Specialist
    c. Anesthesiologist
    d. Urologist

35. Those concerned with the preventing the occurrence of both mental and physical illness and disability is?
    a. Physiatrist
    b. Pathologist
    c. Otolaryngologist
    d. Preventive Medicine Specialist

d. Hantavirus

26. _____ is the principal U.S. federal agency concerned with the health and safety of people throughout the world as his part of HHS?
    a. United Nations
    b. World Health Organization
    c. Centers for Disease Control and Prevention
    d. National Institute of Health

27. Which of this is not a type of health care facility?
    a. Hospital
    b. Ambulatory care
    c. All of the above
    d. None of the above

28. Which of this is not a type of business structure that exists in the medical practice?
    a. Sole Proprietorship
    b. Limited Proprietorship
    c. Partnership
    d. Corporation

29. _____ is defined as an artificial entity having a legal and business status that is independent of its shareholders or employees?
    a. Sole Proprietorship
    b. Limited Proprietorship
    c. Partnership
    d. Corporation

30. Which of the following is the owner potentially liable for all of the acts of his or her professional employees and staff members?
    a. Sole Proprietorship
    b. Limited Proprietorship
    c. Partnership

31. Which of this has the disadvantage where each physician is liable for the actions and conduct of the other?
    a. Sole Proprietorship
    b. Limited Proprietorship
    c. Partnership
    d. Corporation

32. When an individual holds exclusive rights and title to all aspect of the medical practice is called?
    a. Sole Proprietorship
    b. Limited Proprietorship
    c. Partnership
    d. Corporation

33. This specialist uses radioactive substances for the diagnosis and treatment of diseases?
    a. Neurological Surgeon
    b. Nuclear Medicine Specialist
    c. Anesthesiologist
    d. Urologist

34. The medical specialist concerned with the treatment of disease and disorders of the urinary tract is?
    a. Neurological Surgeon
    b. Nuclear Medicine Specialist
    c. Anesthesiologist
    d. Urologist

35. Those concerned with the preventing the occurrence of both mental and physical illness and disability is?
    a. Physiatrist
    b. Pathologist
    c. Otolaryngologist
    d. Preventive Medicine Specialist

36. The physicians that treats diseases and conditions that affects the ears, eyes and throat and structures relating to the head and neck is called?
    a. Thoracic Surgeon
    b. Pathologist
    c. Otolaryngologist
    d. Preventive Medicine Specialist

37. Those concerned with the operative treatment of the chest and chest wall, lungs and respiratory passages are called?
    a. Thoracic Surgeon
    b. Pathologist
    c. Otolaryngologist
    d. Preventive Medicine Specialist

38. The _____ are trained to locate subluxation and remove them using touch and x-ray films thereby restoring the normal flow of nerve energy so that the entire body can function in optimal fashion?
    a. Subluxationist
    b. Nerve Specialist
    c. Chiropractor
    d. Osteopathic

39. The doctor educated in caring for the feet including surgical treatment is called?
    a. Pathologist
    b. Footologist
    c. Dermatologist
    d. Podiatrist

40. Which of this is not a Licensed Medical Professional?
    a. Physician Assistants
    b. Nurse Practitioner
    c. Registered Nurse

41. Which of this is a type of ambulatory care?
    a. Physicians' offices
    b. Group Practices
    c. Multispecialty group
    d. All of the above

42. A type of medicine based on the theory that disturbances in the musculoskeletal system affect other bodily parts causing many disorders that can be corrected by various manipulative techniques in conjunction with conventional medicine surgical and other therapeutic procedures is called?
    a. Chiropractor
    b. Osteopathic
    c. Neurological surgeon
    d. General Surgeon

43. The two major categories of duties of the medical assistance includes?
    a. Receiving and making calls
    b. Filing and retrieving records
    c. Administrative and clinical
    d. None of the above

44. The medical administrative assistant is employed to perform a wide array of duties in various health professions. Which of these is not a major duty?
    a. Management of correspondence
    b. Prepare patient's Bill of Right
    c. Scheduling
    d. Telephone Coverage

45. Which of these areas of medical assistance involves patient contact and assisting physicians in the back office?
    a. Administrative
    b. Health
    c. Assistantship

d. Clinical

46. Which of this is not an area where the Medical assistance can work?
    a. Physician's office
    b. Insurance Companies
    c. Hospitals
    d. None of the above

47. Which of this is an unacceptable behavior for the medical assistance on the externship site?
    a. Handling petty cash in the office
    b. Asking the physician to treat you or family members
    c. Respecting patient's confidentiality
    d. None of the above

48. Which of the following is true about the CMA and RMA?
    a. CMA and RMA certification are awarded by the same agency
    b. CMA and RMA are both nationally recognized certification
    c. All of the above
    d. None of the above

49. Disobedience to authority is known as?
    a. Insubordination
    b. Non-professionalism
    c. Subordination
    d. Improper

50. _____ is defined as exhibiting a courteous, conscientious and generally businesslike manner in the workplace?
    a. Courteousness
    b. Professionalism
    c. Work ethics
    d. Principles

51. Which of this trait alone can influence promotion, termination and the entire atmosphere of the office?
    a. Attitude
    b. Courtesy
    c. Flexibility
    d. Confidentiality

52. What does Work smart mean?
    a. Teamwork
    b. Time management
    c. Using initiative
    d. All of the above

53. Which of this is not a characteristic of professionalism?
    a. Dependability
    b. Flexibility
    c. Credibility
    d. None of the above

54. _____ is an offensive or use of force on a person without his or her consent?
    a. Battery
    b. Offense
    c. Illegal
    d. Defense

55. _____ is the study of the nature, degree and effect if the spatial separation individuals naturally maintain?
    a. Perception
    b. Space
    c. Proxemics
    d. Nonverbal Communication

56. _____ is the process of converting a message into an intelligible form; recognizes and interprets?
    a. Encoding
    b. Decoding
    c. Recording
    d. Interpreting

57. _____ is the process of converting from one system of communication to another; converts a message to a code?
    a. Encoding
    b. Decoding
    c. Recording
    d. Interpreting

58. _____ is the process, function or power of perceiving sounds?
    a. Listening
    b. Speaking
    c. Hearing
    d. Perceiving

59. _____ is defined as paying attention to sound or hearing something with thoughtful attention?
    a. Listening
    b. Speaking
    c. Hearing
    d. Perceiving

60. _____ is the skill whereby paraphrasing and clarifying what the speaker has said take place?
    a. Passive Listening
    b. Active Listening
    c. Paraphrasing
    d. Analyzing

61. _____ is listening to what the sender is communicating, analyzing the words and restating them to confirm that the receiver has understood the message as the sender intended?
    a. Passive Listening
    b. Hearing
    c. Paraphrasing
    d. Analyzing

62. Which form of question is best to ask patients?
    a. Open
    b. Closed
    c. All of the above
    d. None of the above

63. _____ is the reversion to an earlier mental or behavioral level?
    a. Repression
    b. Regression
    c. Rationalization
    d. Suppression

64. The process whereby unwanted desires or impulses are excluded from the consciousness and left to operate in the unconscious is called?
    a. Repression
    b. Regression
    c. Rationalization
    d. Suppression

65. _____ is a lack of feeling, emotion, interest or concern. An indifference to what is happening or a pretense of not caring about a situation?
    a. Repression
    b. Denial
    c. Apathy
    d. Suppression

66. _____ is a psychologic defense mechanism in which confrontation with a personal problem or with reality is avoided by denying the existence of the problem or reality?
    a. Repression
    b. Denial
    c. Apathy
    d. Suppression

67. _____ is defined as the struggle resulting from incompatible or opposing needs, drives, wishes or external or internal demands?
    a. Aggression
    b. Violence
    c. Conflict
    d. Opposition

68. According to Bach in the concept of "crazymaker" which of this is not a characteristic type of passive-aggressive person?
    a. The Attacker
    b. The Trapper
    c. The Avoider
    d. The Mind Reader

69. Instead of allowing their partners to express feelings of honesty the _____ go into character analysis, explaining what the other person really mean or what is wrong with the other person?
    a. The Attacker
    b. The Trapper
    c. The Avoider
    d. The Mind Reader

70. Because they are afraid to face conflicts squarely, the _____ kid around when their partners want to be serious, thus blocking the expression of important feelings?
    a. The Trivial Tyrannizer
    b. The Distractor
    c. The Joker
    d. The Crisis Tickler

71. The _____ brings what is bothering them almost to the surface but never quite expressing their true feelings?
    a. The Trivial Tyrannizer
    b. The Distractor
    c. The Joker
    d. The Crisis Tickler

72. Instead of honestly sharing their resentments, the _____ do things they know will bother their partners?
    a. The Trivial Tyrannizer
    b. The Distractor
    c. The Joker
    d. The Crisis Tickler

73. The _____ will not allow their relationship to change from the way they once were?
    a. The Kitchen sink fighter
    b. The Contract Tyrannizer
    c. The Withholder
    d. TheBeltliner

74. The _____ brings up things that are totally off the subject when in an argument?
    a. The Kitchen sink fighter
    b. The Contract Tyrannizer
    c. The Withholder
    d. The Beltliner

75. Instead of expressing their anger honestly and directly, the _____ punish their partners by holding something back?
    a. The Kitchen sink fighter
    b. The Contract Tyrannizer
    c. The Withholder
    d. The Beltliner

76. _____ is defined as the application of a standardized mental picture that is held in common by members of a group and that represents an oversimplified opinion, prejudiced attitude or uncritical judgment?

   a. Stereotyping
   b. Discrimination
   c. Perception
   d. Prejudice

77. The discernment of what is being communicated according to the message receiver's point of reference is known as?

   a. Stereotyping
   b. Discrimination
   c. Perception
   d. Prejudice

78. Maslow believes that our human needs can be categorized into _____ levels and that the needs on each level must be satisfied before we can move to the next level?

   a. 3
   b. 4
   c. 5
   d. 7

79. On what level does safety and security fall in Maslow's hierarchy of needs?

   a. 1st
   b. 2nd
   c. 3rd
   d. 4th

80. On what level does self-esteem and self-recognition fall in Maslow's hierarchy of needs?
    a. 1st
    b. 2nd
    c. 3rd
    d. 4th

81. Which of this sleep phases are the eyes fairly still and the body relaxes and slows down?
    a. Eye movement
    b. Rapid Eye Movement
    c. Non-Rapid Eye Movement
    d. Deep Sleep

82. Which of this is not a barrier to effective communication?
    a. Physical impairment
    b. Language Differences
    c. Prejudice
    d. None of the above

83. Which level does sleep fall under Maslow's hierarchy of needs?
    a. 1st
    b. 2nd
    c. 3rd
    d. 4th

84. _____ is defined as the thoughts, judgments and actions on issues that have implications of moral right and wrong?
    a. Conduct
    b. Ethics
    c. Principles
    d. Etiquette

85. Refraining from the act of harming or committing evil is called?
    a. Maleficence

b. Nonmaleficence

c. Beneficence

d. Benevolent

86. The act of doing or producing good, especially of performing acts of charity or kindness is?

   a. Maleficence

   b. Nonmaleficence

   c. Beneficence

   d. Favor

87. Faithfulness to something to which one is bounded by pledge or duty is called?

   a. Veracity

   b. Disposition

   c. Fidelity

   d. Benevolence

88. The act or practice of killing or permitting the death of hopelessly sick or injured individuals in a relatively painless way for reason of mercy is?

   a. Euthanasia

   b. Postmortem

   c. Ramifications

   d. Abortion

89. Which of this is not a type of ethical problem presented by Purtilo?

   a. Ethical Distress

   b. Ethical Dilemmas

   c. Dilemmas of Justice

   d. Distress of Justice

90. _____ is a situation in which an individual is faced with two or more choices that are acceptable and correct but doing one thing precludes doing another?

   a. Ethical Distress

   b. Ethical Dilemmas

   c. Dilemmas of Justice

   d. Distress of Justice

91. The type of problem faced when a certain course of action is indicated, but some type of hindrance or barrier prevents that action?
    a. Ethical Distress
    b. Ethical Dilemmas
    c. Dilemmas of Justice
    d. Distress of Justice

92. An intentional, unlawful attempt of bodily injury to another by force is called?
    a. Assault
    b. Battery
    c. Act
    d. Felony

93. Presumed such as when a patient offers an arm for a phlebotomy procedure is called?
    a. Implied consent
    b. Unimplied consent
    c. Informed consent
    d. Uninformed consent

94. A consent usually written which states understanding of what treatment is to be undertaken and of the risk involved, why it should be done and alternative treatment available is called?
    a. Implied consent
    b. Unimplied consent
    c. Informed consent
    d. Uninformed consent

95. A written defamatory statement or representation that conveys an unjust and unfavorable impression is called?
    a. Assault
    b. Slander
    c. Libel
    d. Defamation

96. An oral defamatory; a harmful false statement made about another person is?

   a. Assault
   b. Slander
   c. Libel
   d. Defamation

97. A binding custom or practice of a community; a rule of conduct or action prescribed or formally recognized as binding or enforceable by a controlling authority is called?

   a. Rules
   b. Regulations
   c. Law
   d. Conduct

98. A neutral person chosen to settle differences between two parties in a controversy is?

   a. Appellate
   b. Arbitrator
   c. Jury
   d. 3rd Party

99. A person required to make answer in a legal action or suit, in criminal cases, the person accused of a crime is?

   a. Plaintiff
   b. Defendant
   c. Suspect
   d. Respondent

100. The person required to make answer in a civil legal action or suit is?

   a. Plaintiff
   b. Defendant
   c. Suspect
   d. Respondent

101. Which of this is not a basic category of jurisprudence?

a. Criminal law

b. Civil law

c. Tort law

d. None of the above

102. _____ law governs violations of the law that are punishable as offenses against the state or the government?

a. Criminal law

b. Civil law

c. Tort law

d. Administrative law

103. Which of this is not a basic category of Criminal law?

a. Misdemeanors

b. Felonies

c. Treasons

d. Infractions

104. The offense of attempting to overthrow the government is?

a. Misdemeanors

b. Felonies

c. Treasons

d. Infractions

105. A minor crime punishable by fine or imprisonment in a city or county jail rather than in a penitentiary is?

a. Misdemeanors

b. Felonies

c. Treasons

d. Infractions

106. _____ law provides a remedy for a person or group that has suffered harm from the wrongful act of others?

a. Contract Law

b. Administrative Law

c. Tort Law

d. Justice Law

107. A list of questions from each party to the other in a law suit is?

a. Interrogatories

b. Questioning

c. Inquiring

d. Probing

108. A document issued by a court requiring a person to be in court at a specific time and place to testify as a witness in a lawsuit either in a court proceeding or in a deposition is?

a. Subpoenas

b. Command

c. Order

d. Summon

109. A bench trial is?

a. When the case is open and the defendant is absent

b. When a case is decided by the judge in the absence of a jury

c. When a case is on probation

d. None of the above

110. The performance of an act that is wholly wrongful and unlawful is?

a. Nonfeasance

b. Disfeasance

c. Malfeasance

d. Misfeasance

111. The failure to perform an act that should have been performed is?
    a. Nonfeasance
    b. Disfeasance
    c. Malfeasance
    d. Misfeasance

112. The improper performance of a lawful act is?
    a. Nonfeasance
    b. Disfeasance
    c. Malfeasance
    d. Misfeasance

113. Which of this is not part of the "4 D's of negligence"?
    a. Damage
    b. Danger
    c. Direct cause
    d. Duty

114. Which of the "4 D's of negligence" must there be proof that the harm done to the patient was directly caused by the physicians action or failure to act?
    a. Damage
    b. Danger
    c. Direct cause
    d. Duty

115. Which of the "4 D's of negligence" must the patient proof that a loss or harm has resulted from the actions of the physician?
    a. Damage
    b. Danger
    c. Direct cause
    d. Duty

116. Which of this is not a type of damage seen in tort cases?

    a. Minimal
    b. Special
    c. General
    d. Punitive

117. _____ damages are designed to punish party who committed the wrong in such a way as to deter the repetition of the act?
    a. Compensatory
    b. Special
    c. Nominal
    d. Punitive

118. _____ damages are those injuries or losses that are not a necessary consequence of the physician's negligent act or omission?
    a. Compensatory
    b. Special
    c. General
    d. Punitive

119. Damages that includes compensation for pain and suffering, for loss of a bodily member or faculty, for disfigurement or for other similar direct losses or injuries is?
    a. Compensatory
    b. Special
    c. General
    d. Punitive

120. Exemplary damages can also be called?
    a. Compensatory
    b. Special
    c. General
    d. Punitive

121. A period of time after which a lawsuit cannot be filed is?
    a. Statute of Fraud
    b. Statute of Unfiling

c. Statute of Limitation

d. Statute of Restrain

122. Which of this is not a patient's bill of right?

   a. Respect and Nondiscrimination

   b. Complaints and Appeals

   c. Choice of providers and plans

   d. None of the above

123. Which of this is not a benefit of the HIPAA compliance?

   a. Lowers administrative cost

   b. Increases accuracy of data

   c. Reduces revenue cycle time

   d. None of the above

124. _____ is responsible for the identification of the various hazards present in the workplace and for the creation of rules and regulations to minimize exposure to such hazards?

   a. Employees

   b. Employers

   c. HIPAA

   d. OSHA

125. _____ are mandated to institute measures that will assure safe working conditions and health workers have the obligation to know and follow those measures?

   a. Employees

   b. Employers

   c. HIPAA

   d. OSHA

126. A needle and sharp stick injury log must at a minimum include the following except?

   a. Description of the incident

   b. Type and brand of device used

   c. Time of the incident

d. Location of the incident

127. The hepatitis B Vaccination must be taken by all employees with the first 10days of work for risk of occupational exposure, who is responsible for the cost?
    a. Employees
    b. Employers
    c. CLIA
    d. OSHA

128. For a valid contract to exist there has to be?
    a. A offer
    b. An acceptance
    c. All of the above
    d. None of the above

129. The Americans with Disability Act requires that public medical facilities must allow persons with disabilities to do the following except?
    a. Use drinking fountains, phones and hallways
    b. Do everything that the general public is able to do in the public place
    c. Reach door handles for opening and closing
    d. None of the above

130. Which of this is not a ground for the revocation or suspension of the license to practice medicine?
    a. Personal or professional incapacity
    b. Unprofessional conduct
    c. Conviction of a crime
    d. Arrest

131. Which type of civil law deals with medical professional liability?
    a. Contract Law
    b. Administrative Law
    c. Tort Law
    d. Justice Law

132. Which of this is not an essential element needed for a valid contract?
    a. Manifestation of assent
    b. Contract must involve legal subject matter
    c. Parties to the contract do not need legal capacity to enter into the contract
    d. None of the above

133. Any type of storage of files to prevent their loss in the event of hard disk failure in the future is called?
    a. Backup
    b. Hard disk
    c. Hard drive
    d. Software

134. The smallest units of information inside the computer each represented by either the digit "0" or "1" is?
    a. Kilobyte
    b. Byte
    c. Bite
    d. Bits

135. A unit of data that contains 8 binary digit is?
    a. Kilobyte
    b. Byte
    c. Bite
    d. Bits

136. A device that is capable of "writing" data onto a blank compact disk or copying data from one compact disk to a blank compact is called?
    a. Data writer
    b. CD writer
    c. CD
    d. CD Burner

137. A machine designed to accept, store, process and give out information is?
   a. Printer
   b. Computer
   c. Processor
   d. HP

138. A symbol appearing on the monitor that shows where the next character to be typed will appear is?
   a. Space
   b. Cursor
   c. Line
   d. Margin

139. The nonphysical space appearing of the online world of computer networks in which communication takes place is?
   a. Online space
   b. Cyberspace
   c. Internet space
   d. Nonphysical space

140. A collection of data related files that serves as a foundation for retrieving information is?
   a. Computer
   b. Backup
   c. Database
   d. Microsoft word

141. DVD means?
   a. Digital video drive
   b. Driver video disk
   c. Digital video disk
   d. Disk video drive

142. A removable device shaped like a hard plastic square with a magnetic surface that is capable of storing computer program is?
   a. Disk drives
   b. Hard drive
   c. Disk
   d. DVD

143. Device that loads a program or data stored on a disk into the computer is?
   a. Disk drives
   b. Hard drive
   c. Disk
   d. DVD

144. _____ is also called a diskette?
   a. Disk drive
   b. Hard drive
   c. Disk
   d. DVD

145. An optical disk that holds approximately 28 times more information that a compact disk is?
   a. CD
   b. Hard drive
   c. DVD
   d. Flash Drive

146. Fax is an abbreviation for?
   a. Faxing
   b. Facsimile
   c. Duplicating
   d. Telexing

147. Animation technology used in the opening page of a website to draw attention, excite and impress the user is?
   a. Flash
   b. Animation
   c. Impress
   d. Web design

148. A small portable device that connects into the USB port that can carry 2 to 8 or more gigabytes of information is?
   a. Floppy disk
   b. Zip drive
   c. Flash
   d. Flash drive

149. A small portable disk drive that is primarily used for backing up information and archiving computer files is?
   a. Floppy disk
   b. Zip drive
   c. Flash
   d. Flash drive

150. Approximately 1 billion byte is a?
   a. Megabyte
   b. Kilobyte
   c. Milobyte
   d. Gigabyte

151. Approximately 1 million byte is a?
   a. Megabyte
   b. Kilobyte
   c. Milobyte
   d. Gigabyte

152. A common connecting point for devices in a network containing multiple ports is?
   a. Nub
   b. Port
   c. Hub
   d. Modem

153. HTTP means?
   a. Hyper transfer text protocol
   b. Hyper text transfer protocol
   c. Hyper transfer text processor
   d. Hyper text transfer processor

154. The physical component of the computer is the?
   a. Hardware
   b. Software
   c. Input
   d. Output

155. Pictures often on the desktop of a computer that represent programs or object is?
   a. Media
   b. Picture frame
   c. Programs
   d. Icons

156. MIDI is an acronym for?
   a. Midnight
   b. Midday
   c. Musical Interface Digital Instrument
   d. Musical Instrument Digital Interface

157. A device that allows information to be transmitted over telephone lines at speeds measured in bits per second is?
   a. Nub

b. Server
c. Hub
d. Modem

158. A computer or device on a network that manages shared network resources is?
    a. Router
    b. Server
    c. Hub
    d. Modem

159. A request for information from a database is?
    a. Routing
    b. Queries
    c. Data request
    d. Search engine

160. Information processed by the computer and transmitted to a monitor, printer or other device is?
    a. Hardware
    b. Software
    c. Input
    d. Output

161. Which of this is a basic function of the computer?
    a. Input
    b. Processing
    c. Storage
    d. All of the above

162. The desktop consist of the following except?
    a. Central Processing unit
    b. Mouse
    c. Monitor
    d. None of the above

163. Which of the following devices has embedded computer?
   a. Ultrasound unit
   b. Laptop
   c. Notebook
   d. PDA

164. _____ is the center unit of the computer
   a. Keyboard
   b. CPU
   c. Monitor
   d. Mouse

165. The device used to display computer generated information is the?
   a. Keyboard
   b. CPU
   c. Monitor
   d. Mouse

166. The primary text input of the computer is the?
   a. Keyboard
   b. CPU
   c. Monitor
   d. Mouse

167. _____ is the main circuit board for the computer?
   a. Disk drives
   b. Motherboard
   c. CD-ROM
   d. Memory Card

168. Which of this is not a peripheral device?
   a. Scanners

- b. Digital cameras
- c. Zip drives
- d. Keyboard

169. A computer should be thought of as an additional worker in the office?
- a. True
- b. False
- c. At times
- d. None of the above

170. Which of the following is not a type of printer?
- a. Dot Matrix
- b. Inkjet
- c. Laser
- d. None of the above

171. Telephone calls can be an interruption of the work day for the medical assistant?
- a. True
- b. False
- c. Some times
- d. None of the above

172. When handling the telephone, the mouthpiece should be approximately _____ from the lips?
- a. 1 inch
- b. 0.5 inch
- c. 5 inches
- d. 10 inches

173. After removing the phone from its cradle speak?
- a. After the caller speaks first
- b. After 10 sec
- c. Immediately
- d. As the caller is speaking

174. STAT is an abbreviation for?
   a. Start
   b. Status
   c. System Transmitting at Time
   d. Immediately

175. A change in pitch or loudness of the voice is?
   a. Jargon
   b. Monotone
   c. Diction
   d. Inflection

176. When a patient is inaudible you could use a speakerphone?
   a. True
   b. False
   c. At times
   d. None of the above

177. Never answer a telephone call on the first ring?
   a. True
   b. False
   c. At times
   d. None of the above

178. You can multitask while answering phone calls?
   a. True
   b. False
   c. At times
   d. None of the above

179. It is okay to pick up a phone once it rings and say "please hold" immediately when you are busy?
    a. True
    b. False
    c. At times
    d. None of the above

180. The use of salutation is compulsory in telephone identification?
    a. True
    b. False
    c. At times
    d. None of the above

181. Which of the following is to be considered when scheduling patients for appointment?
    a. Physicians preference and habit
    b. Patient needs
    c. Available facility
    d. All of the above

182. The process of evaluating the urgency of medical need and prioritizing treatment is?
    a. Interval
    b. Intermittent
    c. Triage
    d. Proficiency

183. Coming and going at intervals; not continuous is?
    a. Interval
    b. Intermittent
    c. Triage
    d. Proficiency

184. Competency as a result of training or practice is?
    a. Interval

b. Intermittent

c. Triage

d. Proficiency

185. One disadvantage of computer scheduling is that more than one person cannot access the system at the same time.
   a. True
   b. False
   c. At times
   d. None of the above

186. _____ method of scheduling appointments can also be referred to as tidal wave scheduling?
   a. Wave scheduling
   b. Scheduled Appointment
   c. Double booking
   d. Open office hours

187. Which of this is not a basic feature to consider when choosing an appointment book?
   a. It should be color coded
   b. Size should conform to the desk space
   c. It should open flat for easy writing
   d. It should be large enough to accommodate the practice

188. Something in which a thing originates, develops, takes shape, or is contained; a base on which to build is called?
   a. Integral
   b. Matrix
   c. Expediency
   d. None of the above[

189. The medical administrative should consider the following characteristics when selecting an appointment book except:
   a. Its size in consideration of the amount of desk space available

b. Comfort for writing

c. Number of pages

d. Adequate space for all details necessary

190. When certain number of patients are scheduled to arrive at the same time and are seen in the order in which they arrive is called?
   a. Modified wave scheduling
   b. Modified scheduling
   c. Double Booking
   d. Wave scheduling

191. Scheduling two patients to see the physician at the same time is?
   a. Modified wave scheduling
   b. Modified scheduling
   c. Double Booking
   d. Wave scheduling

192. Small groups of patients are scheduled at intervals throughout the hour is called?
   a. Modified wave scheduling
   b. Modified scheduling
   c. Double Booking
   d. Wave scheduling

193. The Medical Administrative Assistant should do the following when scheduling a new patient except
   a. The Medical Assistant can schedule appointment time for patient solely in his/her discretion without the patient's consent
   b. Gather appropriate information regarding a patient referral
   c. Determine the proper financial arrangements for the patient's appointment
   d. Determine the patient's chief complaint

194. The Medical Administrative Assistant should do the following when scheduling an established patient except:
   a. Gather the appropriate information in order to properly identify the patient

b. Do without verification of information since they are established patient

c. Provide patient with appointment card if necessary

d. Enter the appropriate time for the appointment

195. Which of this is not a way in which the medical assistant can help prepare a patient for an examination?

   a. Escort patient to the examination room and other areas of the office

   b. Make sure that the patients wallet and other items are secured

   c. Stay with the patient all through the examination and after

   d. Ask whether the patient has any questions

196. The following are ways to make patient feel at ease and comfortable in the medical office except?

   a. Personal touch

   b. Attractive reception

   c. Using the patient's name often

   d. None of the above

197. A person who comes to a country to take up permanent residence is called?

   a. Permanent Resider

   b. Green card holder

   c. Immigrant

   d. Migrant

198. A two way communication system with a microphone and loudspeaker at each station for localized used is?

   a. Headset

   b. Handset

   c. Intercom

   d. Starcom

199. Notes used in the patient chart to track the progress and condition of the patient is called?

   a. Progress notes

b. Patient chart book

c. Patient file

d. Patient record

200. The statistical characteristics of human populations used especially to identify markets is called?

   a. Statistical data

   b. Population census

   c. Demographic

   d. All of the above

201. An accounting period of 12 months during which a company determines earnings and profit is called?

   a. Annual year

   b. Fiscal year

   c. Profit sharing year

   d. None of the above

202. The practice of subcontracting work to an outside company is called?

   a. Delegation

   b. Subcontracting

   c. Designating

   d. Outsourcing

203. Differences amongst conflicting facts, claims or opinions is called?

   a. Differentiation

   b. Discrepancies

   c. Variety

   d. Diversity

204. Marking a document or a specific place within a document for later retrieval; a feature supported by most browsers that allows user to save the address so that the document can be located when it is needed again is?

   a. Bookmark

b. History

c. Backmark

d. Saving document

205. An order item that has not been delivered when promised or demanded but will be supplied at a later date is?

a. Backorder

b. Backlog

c. None Delivery

d. Failed promise

206. A plan for the coordination of resources and expenditures; the amount of money that is available or required for a particular purpose is?

a. Planning

b. Organizing

c. Budget

d. Revenue

207. A list of items that are included in a shipment is called?

a. Shipment slip

b. Packing slip

c. Item list

d. Invoice

208. To become liable or subject to; to bring down on oneself is called?

a. Humility

b. Liability

c. Self-esteem

d. Incur

209. Acting in anticipation of future problems, needs or changes is?
   a. Action
   b. Inaction
   c. Proactive
   d. All of the above

210. When moving through hallways, the medical assistance should walk on the?
   a. Left side
   b. Right side
   c. Middle
   d. Anywhere

211. The office policy manual should be read?
   a. When the medical assistant begin work at the physician's office
   b. As a daily source of information for all employees to reference whenever needed
   c. At least annually
   d. All of the above

212. The office policy manual should include the following except?
   a. Sexual harassment
   b. Vacations
   c. Continuing education
   d. Pay scale

213. Below are some expenses that are involved in the operation of a medical practice except?
   a. Taxes
   b. Utilities
   c. Medical equipment
   d. Legal expenses

214. An itemized list of goods shipped that specifies price and the term of sale is?
   a. Invoice
   b. Bill

c. Statement

d. Receipt

215. A statement of financial account that shows the balance due as well as transactions that affects the account is?

    a. Invoice
    b. Bill
    c. Statement
    d. Receipt

216. The following are ways in which physician's office employees can reduce waste while saving money except?

    a. Use solar powered calculators and batter rechargers
    b. Use refillable pens and pencils
    c. Use bulletin board
    d. None of the above

217. In the case of a robbery, the medical assistance should make every effort to remember the following basic identification markers except?

    a. Hand
    b. Weight
    c. Race
    d. Clothing

218. For office security the alarm code should be known by?

    a. All staff members
    b. Only the office manager
    c. Only Physician
    d. The office manager and those who open and close the facility and physician

219. The use of fire extinguisher can be memorized using the mnemonics device PASS; the "P" means?

    a. Please

b. Pull the pin

c. Point of pulling

d. Place to pull

220. The use of fire extinguisher can be memorized using the mnemonics device PASS; the "A" means?

    a. Act

    b. Action

    c. Aim the hose

    d. Arm the hose

221. The use of fire extinguisher can be memorized using the mnemonics device PASS; the first "S" means?

    a. Seize the nozzle

    b. Squeeze

    c. Sweep the nozzle

    d. Strip

222. The use of fire extinguisher can be memorized using the mnemonics device PASS; the second "S" means?

    a. Seize the nozzle

    b. Squeeze

    c. Sweep the nozzle

    d. Strip

223. _____ is the applied science concerned with designing and arranging things people use so that the people and the things interact efficiently and safely?

    a. Ergonomics

    b. Acoustics

    c. White Noise

    d. Audibility

224. _____ is defined as the science that deals with the production, control, transmission, reception, and effects of sound?

a. Ergonomics

b. Acoustics

c. White Noise

d. Audibility

225. The following actions are needed to be taken before the office opens in the morning except?

   a. Office should be clean

   b. Make two copies of the appointment book

   c. Phones should be turned to answering machine

   d. Exam room supplies should be checked and replaced when necessary

226. A durable, formal paper used for document is?

   a. Typing sheet

   b. A4 paper

   c. Bond

   d. Formal paper

227. Method of payment used when an article or item is delivered and payment is expected before released is?

   a. Collect on delivery

   b. Payment on delivery

   c. Delivered on payment

   d. All of the above

228. The receiver of something or item is?

   a. Acceptor

   b. Collector

   c. Recipient

   d. Heir

229. A marking in paper resulting from differences in thickness usually produced by the pressure of a projecting design in the mold or on a processing roll and visible when the paper is held up to the light is?

a. Bookmark
b. Watermark
c. Papermark
d. Design mark

230. Furnishing with notes that are usually critical or explanatory is?
a. Annotating
b. Noting
c. Appendix
d. Glossary

231. Which of the nouns are specific?
a. Common noun
b. Proper noun
c. Pronoun
d. Specific noun

232. Connecting words that shows a relationship between nouns, pronouns or other words in a sentence are called?
a. Adverb
b. Adjective
c. Preposition
d. Conjunction

233. Which of the following is not a part of speech?
a. Verb
b. Sentence
c. Noun
d. Preposition

234. Which of the following is not a type of sentence?
a. Declarative
b. Imperative
c. Statement

d. Exclamatory

235. Which of this type of sentence states a command or request?
a. Declarative
b. Imperative
c. Statement
d. Exclamatory

236. Which of the following is not a basic pattern for constructing sentence?
a. Subject predicate
b. Subject object
c. Subject complement
d. None of the above

237. _____ is an incomplete thought or a portion of a sentence that is punctuated as though it were a complete sentence?
a. Run on sentence
b. Sentence fragment
c. Comma splice
d. Subject predicate

238. The part of a sentence that contains the verb and tells what the subject is doing or experiencing or what is being done to the subject is?
a. Run on sentence
b. Sentence fragment
c. Comma splice
d. Subject predicate

239. A sentence that contains independent clauses without a semicolon or comma between them is called?

   a. Run on sentence
   b. Sentence fragment
   c. Comma splice
   d. Subject predicate

240. _____ type of sentence is also called run-together?

   a. Run on sentence
   b. Sentence fragment
   c. Comma splice
   d. Subject predicate

241. When writing letter in a block letter style where should you have your signature located?

   a. Top Right
   b. Lower Right
   c. Lower middle
   d. Lower Left

242. When writing letter in a modified block letter style where should you have your signature located?

   a. Top Right
   b. Lower Right
   c. Lower middle
   d. Lower Left

243. Which of the following numbers will be filled Second?

   a. 4321234
   b. 4123453
   c. 3487631
   d. 4123443

244. Which of this names will be filled Third?

a. Adam-Smith
b. Adams
c. Adamu
d. Anna

245. First-class mail that weighs more than 13 ounces is called?
a. Priority Mail
b. Express Mail
c. Certified Mail
d. Bulk Mailing

246. This type of mail is available every day of the year, including holidays, for items up to 70 lbs in weight and 108 inches in height
a. Priority Mail
b. Express Mail
c. Certified Mail
d. Bulk Mailing

247. This type of mailing gives the sender the option to receive proof of delivery?
a. Media Mail
b. Express Mail
c. Certified Mail
d. First class Mail

248. This type of mail includes letters, postal cards, postcards, and business reply mail?
a. Media Mail
b. Express Mail
c. First class Mail
d. Certified Mail

249. _____ is used for books, films, manuscripts, printed music, printed test materials, videotapes and computer recorded media
a. Media Mail

b. Express Mail

c. First class Mail

d. Certified Mail

250. Which of the following is not a basic size of envelop?

a. No. 10

b. No. 5

c. No. 6 ¾

d. Window

MA Test 1

1	C
2	D
3	B
4	A
5	C
6	C
7	C
8	A
9	B
10	A
11	D
12	A
13	B
14	D
15	B
16	A
17	B
18	C
19	B
20	B
21	D
22	D
23	B
24	C
25	A
26	C
27	D
28	B

29	D
30	A
31	C
32	A
33	B
34	D
35	D
36	C
37	A
38	C
39	D
40	D
41	D
42	B
43	C
44	B
45	D
46	D
47	B
48	B
49	A
50	B
51	A
52	B
53	D
54	A
55	C
56	B
57	A
58	C
59	A
60	B
61	C
62	A
63	B
64	A
65	C
66	B
67	C
68	A
69	D
70	C
71	D
72	A
73	B

74	A
75	C
76	A
77	C
78	C
79	B
80	D
81	C
82	D
83	A
84	B
85	B
86	C
87	C
88	A
89	D
90	B
91	A
92	A
93	A
94	C
95	C
96	B
97	C
98	B
99	B
100	D
101	C
102	A
103	D
104	C
105	A
106	C
107	A
108	A
109	B
110	C
111	A
112	D
113	B
114	C
115	A
116	A
117	D
118	B

119	C
120	D
121	C
122	D
123	D
124	D
125	B
126	C
127	B
128	C
129	D
130	D
131	C
132	C
133	A
134	D
135	B
136	D
137	B
138	B
139	B
140	C
141	C
142	C
143	A
144	C
145	C
146	B
147	A
148	D
149	B
150	D
151	A
152	C
153	B
154	A
155	D
156	D
157	D
158	B
159	B
160	D
161	D
162	D
163	A

#	Answer
164	B
165	C
166	A
167	B
168	D
169	A
170	D
171	B
172	A
173	C
174	D
175	D
176	B
177	B
178	B
179	B
180	B
181	D
182	C
183	B
184	D
185	B
186	D
187	A
188	B
189	C
190	D
191	C
192	A
193	A
194	B
195	C
196	D
197	C
198	C
199	A
200	C
201	B
202	D
203	B
204	A
205	A
206	C
207	B
208	D

209	C
210	B
211	D
212	D
213	D
214	A
215	C
216	C
217	A
218	D
219	B
220	C
221	B
222	C
223	A
224	B
225	C
226	C
227	A
228	C
229	B
230	A
231	B
232	C
233	B
234	C
235	B
236	D
237	B
238	D
239	A
240	A
241	D
242	C
243	D
244	C
245	A
246	B
247	C
248	C
249	A
250	B

Review Questions 2

1. Which of this is not a reason for the existence of medical records?

    a. Assist physician in providing the best possible medical care for the patient

    b. Provides statistical information that is helpful to researchers

    c. Vital for financial reimbursement

    d. None of the above

2. Who owns the medical record?

    a. Patient

    b. Physician

    c. Patient's sponsor

    d. Insurance Company

3. Adopting a medical record management system that works in other facilities is the best as it saves time and you are sure it will work?

    a. True

    b. False

    c. At times

    d. None of the above

4. Which of this is not a major type of patient's medical record?

    a. Paper-based

    b. Computer-based

c. Objective-based

d. None of the above

5. Which of the following is also called the "electronic health record"?

    a. Paper-based

    b. Computer-based

    c. Objective-based

    d. Subjective-based

6. In the organization of the medical record, which of this is seen as the traditional patient record?

    a. Problem oriented medical record

    b. SOAP

    c. Source oriented

    d. None of the above

7. Which of the following is sometimes referred to as the "weed system"?

    a. Problem oriented medical record

    b. SOAP

    c. Source oriented

    d. None of the above

8. The "S" in SOAP is an acronym for?

    a. Start

    b. Shingling

    c. Subjective

    d. Selection

9. The "O" in SOAP is an acronym for?

    a. Objection

    b. Order

    c. Oriented

    d. Objective

10. The "A" in SOAP is an acronym for?

    a. Assessment

    b. Align

    c. Adapt

    d. Alignment

11. The "P" in SOAP is an acronym for?

    a. Problem

    b. Plan

    c. Prepare

    d. Prognosis

12. Information gained by questioning the patient or taken from a form is known as?

    a. Subjective Information

    b. Objective Information

    c. Computer Based

    d. Paper Based

13. Information that is gathered by watching or observing of a patient is?

a. Subjective Information

b. Objective Information

c. Computer Based

d. Paper Based

14. Which of this is not a subjective information?

    a. Personal Demographics

    b. Patient's family history

    c. Patient's chief complaint

    d. Diagnosis

15. The Medical Administrative Assistant should take the following steps to establish a patient's medical record except:

    a. Determine the patient's status in the office

    b. Enter the patient's name into the computerized ledger

    c. Assemble the appropriate forms, prepare the folder and file as necessary

    d. All of the Above

16. A decision made based on the information regarding the patient's history and the results of the doctor's examination is called

    a. Prognosis

    b. Diagnosis

    c. Patient's chief complaint

    d. All of the above

17. Medical record created using information like past illnesses, surgical operations, and the patient's daily health habits gathered from the patient is known as:

    a. Patient's Family History

    b. Patient's Social History

    c. Diagnosis

    d. Personal and Medical History

18. When making corrections to a medical record which of this is appropriate to do?

    a. Erase using Correction fluid

    b. Rewrite on the Error

    c. Draw a line through the error and insert the correction above

    d. All of the above

19. After all medical records has been reviewed for the day, if it is impossible to be filed before the close of day, it should be?

    a. Placed in a file tray and locked away

    b. Left on the medical assistant table as a reminder to be filed the next day

    c. Put on the Physician's table

    d. Any of the above

20. Which of this is not a filing classification of records?

    a. Open

    b. Closed

    c. Active

    d. Inactive

21. When no restriction exist for retention of medical record, it is best the record be kept for a period of?

   a. 5 months
   b. 5 years
   c. 1 year
   d. 10 years

22. When a patient decides that he or she no longer agrees to release medical information to third party, which of this form does he need to sign?

   a. Non-release form
   b. Retention form
   c. Revocation form
   d. All of the above

23. Which of this is not involved in the process of dictations and transcription?

   a. Dictating into a dictation unit
   b. Listening to what has been dictated
   c. Keyboarding dictated text to a printed document
   d. None of the above

24. Which of this is not a consideration in selecting filing equipment?

   a. Availability of office space
   b. Color of cabinet
   c. Size and volume of record
   d. Retrieval speed

25. Which of the following is the most economic but offer little protection or confidentiality to the records?

   a. Drawer files

   b. Shelf files

   c. Rotary circular files

   d. Lateral files

26. When some marks are placed on the paper indicating that it is now ready for filing is called?

   a. Bookmark

   b. File mark

   c. Releasing

   d. Ready filing

27. _____ means deciding where to file letters or paper?

   a. Coding

   b. Indexing

   c. Conditioning

   d. Releasing

28. _____ means placing some indication of the decision on where to file on the paper?

   a. Coding

   b. Indexing

   c. Conditioning

   d. Releasing

29. When storing or filing papers in the folder, items should be placed?

   a. Face down

   b. Face up

   c. Top edge to the right

   d. Any of the above

30. In filing, the middle name comes?

   a. Middle

   b. First

   c. Second

   d. Third

31. In filing, the last name comes?

   a. Last

   b. First

   c. Second

   d. Third

32. In filing which of the following should come second?

   a. John-Doe Smith

   b. Jason Jackson

   c. Zee Zig

   d. Peter Street

33. How should the name John-Doe Smith be filed?

    a. Doe John Smith

    b. John Doe Smith

    c. Smith, Johndoe

    d. John-Doe Smith

34. The three basic methods of filing in healthcare facilities are as follows except?

    a. Alphabetic

    b. Numeric

    c. Color coding

    d. Subject

35. Which of the following has a direct filing system?

    a. Alphabetic

    b. Numeric

    c. Color coding

    d. Subject

36. Which of the following has an indirect filing system?

    a. Alphabetic

    b. Numeric

    c. Color coding

    d. Subject

37. Which of the following filing can either be alphabetic or alphanumeric?

a. Alphabetic

b. Numeric

c. Color coding

d. Subject

38. _____ file is used for materials that have no permanent value?

    a. Transitory file

    b. Practice management file

    c. Tickler file

    d. Follow up file

39. A filing system in which materials can be located without consulting an intermediary source of reference is?

    a. Direct filing system

    b. Indirect filing system

    c. Intermediary filing system

    d. Non intermediary filing system

40. A filing system in which an intermediary source of reference must be consulted to locate specific files is?

    a. Direct filing system

    b. Indirect filing system

    c. Intermediary filing system

    d. Non intermediary filing system

41. A film bearing a photographic record on a reduced scale of printed or other graphic matter is?

    a. Photographic film

b. Graphic film

c. Micro film

d. Reduce scale film

42. A folder used to provide space for the temporary filing of materials is?

   a. Temporary file

   b. Transitory folder

   c. OUTfolder

   d. OUTguide

43. A heavy guide that is used to replace a folder that has been temporarily moved from the filing space is?

   a. Temporary file

   b. Transitory folder

   c. OUTfolder

   d. OUTguide

44. A temporary diagnosis made before all test result have been received is?

   a. Provisional diagnosis

   b. Prognosis

   c. Projectional diagnosis

   d. Temporary diagnosis

45. Which of this is not one of the 9 characteristics of quality health care?

   a. Timeliness

   b. Openness

c. Relevance

d. Security

46. In 1996 _____ was developed to help ensure the confidentiality of medical record?

   a. HIPAA

   b. NCHS

   c. JCAHO

   d. None of the above

47. Which of the following is a nonprofit organization that assist healthcare facilities provide accreditation services?

   a. HIPAA

   b. NCHS

   c. JCAHO

   d. None of the above

48. _____ is any occurrence that could result in patient injury any type of financial loss to the healthcare facility?

   a. Carelessness

   b. Procrastination

   c. Risk

   d. Hazard

49. An unexpected occurrence involving death or serious physical or psychological injury or the risk thereof is?

a. Sentinel event

   b. Unexpected event

   c. Force major

   d. Unexpected risk

50. Activities designed to increase the quality of a product or service through process or system changes that increases efficiency and effectiveness is called?

   a. Activity changes

   b. Efficiency improvement

   c. Continuous improvement

   d. Quality Assurance

51. Title II provision of the HIPAA deals with?

   a. Insurance Reform

   b. Administrative simplification

   c. Healthcare reforms

   d. Federal government laws

52. Title II provision of the HIPAA deals with?

   a. Insurance Reform

   b. Administrative simplification

   c. Healthcare reforms

   d. Federal government laws

53. Individuals or organizations that perform or assist a covered entity in the performance of a function or activity that involves the use or disclosure of individually identifiable health information is?

    a. Business associates

    b. Individual health information coverage

    c. Business health information coverage

    d. All of the above

54. A person making a complaint against a person or organisation is known as _____?

    a. Complainer

    b. Chief complaint

    c. Complainant

    d. Accuser

55. _____ is also known as due care?

    a. Divulge

    b. Appropriate care

    c. Due Diligence

    d. Required care

56. The effort made by an ordinary prudent or reasonable party to avoid harm to another party or himself is?

    a. Divulge

    b. Appropriate care

    c. Due Diligence

    d. Required care

57. Providers of medical or health services, individually or as organizations, that furnish, bill for or are paid for services or products is?

   a. Hospitals

   b. Health facilities

   c. Healthcare providers

   d. Medicare

58. To derive conclusion from facts and premises is called?

   a. Hypothesis

   b. Infer

   c. Concluding fact

   d. Assumption

59. The division of the federal government that enforces privacy standards is called?

   a. Office of the privacy standard act

   b. Office of Inspector General

   c. Office for Health information Enforcement

   d. Office for Civil Rights

60. The patient's own information that pertains to his or her health is called?

   a. Patient's information

   b. Private information

   c. Personal health information

   d. All of the above

61. A person designated to ensure compliance with privacy standards for a covered entity is?

   a. Compliance officer

   b. Submission officer

   c. Privacy officer

   d. All of the above

62. Transmission of information between two parties to carry out financial or administrative activies related to healthcare is?

   a. Medical assistance

   b. Transmissionist

   c. Information transmission

   d. Transactions

63. _____ is established to protect the integrity of the department of health and human services, the office conduct audits, investigation and inspection involving laws that pertains to HHS?

   a. Office of Investigation and Inspection Audit

   b. Office of Inspector General

   c. Office for Health information Enforcement

   d. Office for Civil Rights

64. When a patient has a complaint regarding his or her privacy information, the first person he should seek out is the?

   a. Office Manager
   b. Privacy officer
   c. Office for Civil Rights
   d. Office of the Inspector General

65. Which of the following must be included on a notice of privacy practices?

   a. Details of how PHI is used and disclosed by the facility
   b. Duties of providers to protect health information
   c. Effective date of the notice of privacy practice
   d. All of the above

66. Which of this is not a right that the patient has under privacy rule?

   a. Right to request that communication from the facility be kept confidential
   b. Right to charge a physician if he is not satisfied with his service
   c. Right to restrict certain parts or uses of their PHI
   d. Right to notice of a facility's privacy practice

67. _____ is a secondary use or disclosure that cannot reasonably be prevented, it is limited in nature and occurs as a result of another use or disclosure that is permitted?

   a. Secondary Disclosure
   b. Primary Disclosure
   c. Permitted Disclosure
   d. Incidental Disclosure

68. Services that support patient diagnoses is called?

    a. Ancillary therapeutic services

    b. Patient diagnoses services

    c. Patient treatment services

    d. Ancillary diagnostic services

69. Services that support patient treatment is called?

    a. Ancillary therapeutic services

    b. Patient diagnoses services

    c. Patient treatment services

    d. Ancillary diagnostic services

70. Converting verbal or written descriptions into numeric and alphanumeric designations is called?

    a. Filing

    b. Coding

    c. Converting

    d. Transforming

71. The determination of the nature of disease, injury, or congenital defect is?

    a. Determinant

    b. Prognosis

    c. Porosis

    d. Diagnosis

72. The acronym ICD-9-CM means?

    a. International clinical data, Ninth Revision Classification Modification

    b. Internal Classification of Disease Non Revised Clinical Modification

    c. International Classification of Diseases Ninth Revision, Clinical Modification

    d. None of the above

73. System containing the greatest number of changes in ICD history to allow specific reporting of disease and newly recognized conditions is?

    a. ICD-9-CM

    b. ICD-5-CM

    c. ICD-11-CM

    d. ICD-10-CM

74. System for classifying disease to facilitate the collection of uniform and comparable health information, for statistical purposes and indexing medical records for data storage and retrieval is called?

    a. ICD-9-CM

    b. ICD-5-CM

    c. ICD-11-CM

    d. ICD-10-CM

75. The initial identification of the condition or complaint that the patient expresses in the outpatient medical setting?

    a. Chief Complaint

    b. Initial Complaint

    c. Patient Identification

d. Primary Diagnosis

76. The ICD-10-CM contains approximately _____ more codes that ICD-9.

    a. 5000

    b. 4500

    c. 5500

    d. 6500

77. The translation and transformation of written descriptions of diseases, illness and injury into numeric codes is called?

    a. Classification of diseases

    b. Diagnostic coding

    c. Descriptive numeric coding

    d. None of the above

78. The ICD-9-CM manuals contains three volumes, Volumes 1 & 2 are used for?

    a. Coding procedures and services performed within hospital environment

    b. V coding

    c. E coding

    d. Diagnostic coding

79. The ICD-9-CM manuals contains three volumes, Volume 3 is used for?

    a. Coding procedures and services performed within hospital environment

    b. V coding

    c. E coding

130

d. Diagnostic coding

80. Volume 1 of the ICD-9-CM manual is also known as the?

   a. Tabular Index

   b. Numeric Index

   c. Alphabetic Index

   d. Alphanumeric Index

81. The _____ code classification is named the supplemental classification of external causes of injuries and poisoning?

   a. V coding

   b. A coding

   c. E coding

   d. Procedural coding

82. Volume 2 of the ICD-9-CM manual is called the?

   a. Tabular Index

   b. Numeric Index

   c. Alphabetic Index

   d. Alphanumeric Index

83. The _____ code is used on occasions when the patient is not currently ill or to explain problems that influence his current illness?

   a. V code

   b. A code

c. E code

d. Procedural coding

84. The _____ code is used to classify environmental causes of injury, poisoning or other adverse effect on the body?

   a. V code

   b. A code

   c. E code

   d. Procedural coding

85. The abbreviation "NOS" used on the tabular index of the ICD-9-CM means?

   a. Numbers

   b. Not on site

   c. Number of Sickness

   d. Not otherwise specified

86. The abbreviation "NEC" used on the tabular index of the ICD-9-CM means?

   a. Number of etiology classification

   b. Not excluding category

   c. Not elsewhere classifiable

   d. No external classification

87. Which of the volumes of the ICD-9-CM manual is not used in a physician's office?

   a. Volume 1

   b. Volume 2

   c. Volume 3

d. None of the above

88. _____ is a residual problem remaining after acute phase of an illness or injury has terminated?

   a. Suspected
   b. Late effect
   c. Impending threat
   d. Parasitic Diseases

89. _____ refers to the underlying cause or origin of a disease?

   a. Manifestation
   b. Etiology
   c. Root cause
   d. Indicators

90. _____ describes the signs and symptoms of a disease?

   a. Manifestation
   b. Etiology
   c. Root cause
   d. Indicators

91. In coding, the circulatory system section for *hypertensive disease* can be found in category?

   a. 393 to 398
   b. 415 to 417
   c. 420 to 429

d. 390 to 392

92. In coding, the circulatory system section for acute *rheumatic fever* can be found in category?

   a. 393 to 398

   b. 415 to 417

   c. 420 to 429

   d. 390 to 392

93. _____ is caused by a lesion on one of the coronary arteries that causes lack of blood flow to the heart?

   a. Myocardial Infarction

   b. Hypertension disease

   c. Ischemic heart disease

   d. Cerebrovascular accident

94. _____ is defined as the transformation of verbal descriptions of medical services and procedures into numeric or alphanumeric designations?

   a. Diagnostic coding

   b. Procedural coding

   c. CPT-4 manual

   d. HCPCS

95. A listing of descriptive terms and identifying codes for reporting medical services and procedures performed by physicians in order to provide a uniform or standard language that will accurately

describe medical, surgical and diagnostic services and enhance reliable communication among physician is?

    a. Diagnostic coding

    b. Procedural coding

    c. CPT-4 manual

    d. HCPCS

96. Code additions that explain circumstances that alter a provided service or provide additional clarification or detail about a procedure or service is?

    a. Additional service codes

    b. Procedural code

    c. Modifiers

    d. All of the above

97. Codes in which the components of a procedure are separated and reported separately is?

    a. Subcategory code

    b. Bundled code

    c. Subsection code

    d. Unbundled code

98. Codes designating procedures or services that are grouped together and paid for as one procedure or service is?

    a. Subcategory code

    b. Bundled code

    c. Subsection code

    d. Unbundled code

99. The primary procedure or service code selected when performing insurance billing or statistical research is?

   a. Subcategory
   b. Category I code
   c. Category II code
   d. Category III code

100. Indented one level below a category, usually a procedure or service unique to a category is?

   a. Subcategory
   b. Category I code
   c. Category II code
   d. Category III code

101. Code for a new experimental procedure or service is called?

   a. Subcategory
   b. Category I code
   c. Category II code
   d. Category III code

102. Special codes that can help providers track revenue and reimbursement is?

   a. Subcategory
   b. Category I code
   c. Category II code
   d. Category III code

103. A patient is diagnosed with metastatic bone neoplasm. The neoplasm will be coded as?

a. Primary malignant

b. Secondary malignant

c. Carcinoma in situ

d. Benign

104. _____ is defined as the absence of invasion of surrounding tissues.

a. Primary malignant

b. Secondary malignant

c. Carcinoma in situ

d. Benign

105. The _____ code is used for procedures that is always performed during the same operative session as another surgery in addition to the primary service/procedure and is never performed separately?

a. Stand-alone codes

b. Indented codes

c. Add-on codes

d. Modifiers

106. _____ is used when more than one code must be used to completely describe a specific procedure or service?

a. Circle with a line through it

b. Two triangular symbols

c. A bullet

d. A plus sign

107. _____ represents a new procedure or service code added/revised since the previous edition of the CPT manual?

   a. Circle with a line through it

   b. Two triangular symbols

   c. A bullet

   d. A plus sign

108. The _____ are reported as two-digit numeric codes added to the five-digit CPT code?

   a. Modifiers

   b. Add-on codes

   c. Location Method

   d. All of the above

109. All of the following are correct regarding add-on codes except:

   a. They can be reported as stand-alone codes.

   b. They are exempted from modifier-51 (multiple procedures).

   c. They are performed in addition to a primary procedure.

   d. The add-on procedure must be performed by the same physician

110. What are the three key components of an E & M Code?

   a. Examination, coordination of care, medical decision making

   b. History, examination, medical decision making

   c. History, nature of presenting problem, coordination of care

   d. Nature of presenting problem, examination, coordination of care

138

111. If a code is selected that not only matches the procedure or service performed but also add modifying information that is not in the medical documentation, the information is considered _____?

   a. Downcoding

   b. Noncoding

   c. Upcoded

   d. Modifying codes

112. _____ are procedures or services named after their inventor or developer?

   a. Eponyms

   b. Scientist

   c. Mohs

   d. Crohn

113. A change in code submitted to reimbursement usually performed by the insurance company is called?

   a. Downcoding

   b. Noncoding

   c. Upcoded

   d. Modifying codes

114. Which of the following is not a category in which the E&M section is divided into?

   a. Office visits

   b. Hospital visits

   c. Consultations

   d. None of the above

115. A new patient is?

- a. One who has not visited the physician in more than 6 months
- b. One who has not been seen by any of the physicians in 3 years.
- c. Determined by the physician and staff
- d. Determined by a third-party payer

116. _____ is defined as someone who has received medical services within the last 3 years from the physician or another physician of the same specialty who belongs to the same group practice?

- a. New patient
- b. Established patient
- c. Old patient
- d. Returning patient

117. _____ is a brief statement describing the symptom, problem, diagnosis, or condition that is the reason a patient seeks medical care?

- a. Prognosis
- b. Patient medical history
- c. Chief complaint
- d. Prescription

118. Which of the following is not a circumstance under which the V codes are used?

- a. To indicate the birth status of a newborn
- b. When a circumstance may influence a patient's health status but is not a current illness or condition

c. When a person has virus that has not yet been cured

d. When a person who is not currently sick encounters the health services for some specific reason such as to act as an organ donor or receive a vaccination

119. The _____ codes are used to describe the reason or external cause of injury?

   a. Volume 1
   b. E code
   c. V code
   d. All of the above

120. The Abbreviation "POS" means?

   a. Position
   b. Post out of service
   c. Possible outcome solution
   d. Point of service

121. When the patient answers questions about the eyes, ears, nose, throat and mouth it is called?

   a. Chief complaint
   b. Past medical and social history
   c. Review of systems
   d. History of present illness

122. _____ concentrates on the chief complaint, it looks at the symptoms, severity and duration of problem?

   a. Problem focused history

b. Detailed history

c. Expanded problem focused history

d. Comprehensive history

123. When the physician proceeds as in the problem focused history but includes a review of the system that refers to chief complaint is?

   a. Problem focused history

   b. Detailed history

   c. Expanded problem focused history

   d. Comprehensive history

124. Which of this is not a division in examination in the evaluation and management service?

   a. Detailed examination

   b. Expanded problem focused examination

   c. Comprehensive examination

   d. None of the above

125. In anesthesia coding, the physical status modifiers is composed of two characters, "P1" represents?

   a. A normal healthy patient

   b. A brain-dead patient whose organ are being harvested

   c. A patient with severe systemic disease

   d. A patient with mild systemic disease

126. In anesthesia coding, the physical status modifiers is composed of two characters, "P2" represents?

   a. A normal healthy patient
   b. A brain-dead patient whose organ are being harvested
   c. A patient with severe systemic disease
   d. A patient with mild systemic disease

127. In anesthesia coding, the physical status modifiers is composed of two characters, "P5" represents?

   a. A normal healthy patient
   b. A brain-dead patient whose organ are being harvested
   c. A patient with severe systemic disease
   d. A patient with mild systemic disease

128. _____ codes are intended to report a hydration intravenous infusion to consist of a prepackaged fluid and electrolytes but are not used to report infusion of drugs or other substance?

   a. Psychotherapy
   b. Vaccines
   c. Toxoids
   d. Hydration

129. _____ is the treatment for mental illness and behavioral disturbance in which he clinical attempts to alleviate the emotional disturbances, reverse or change maladaptive patters of behavior and encourages personality growth and development?

   a. Psychotherapy
   b. Vaccines

c. Toxoids

d. Hydration

130. _____ codes are reported once per month to distinguish age specific service related to the patient's end stage renal disease performed in an outpatient setting?

   a. Psychotherapy

   b. Dialysis

   c. Toxoids

   d. Hydration

131. _____ is an ultrasound examination of the cardiac chambers and calves, the adjacent great vessels, and the pericardium?

   a. Cardiac catheterization

   b. Echocardiography

   c. Chemotherapy

   d. Electrophysiology

132. A diagnostic medical procedure that includes introduction, positioning and repositioning of catheter, recording of intracardiac and intravascular pressure and final evaluation and reporting of the procedure is?

   a. Cardiac catheterization

   b. Echocardiography

   c. Chemotherapy

   d. Electrophysiology

133. The continuous and simultaneous monitoring and recording of various physiologic parameters of sleep for 6 or more hours with physician review, interpretation and report is?

   a. Sleep monitoring

   b. Physiologic parameters of sleep

   c. Sleep studies

   d. All of the above

134. An injection in which the healthcare professional who administers the substance or drugs is continuously present to administer the injection and observe the patient or an infusion of 15 minutes or less is?

   a. Intraarterial push

   b. Injection observation

   c. Acupuncture

   d. All of the above

135. _____ procedures are performed to remove devitalized and necrotic tissue and promote healing?

   a. Acupuncture

   b. Active wound care

   c. Osteopathic Manipulative

   d. Home health procedures

136. _____ is reported based on 15 minutes increments of personal contact with patient?

   a. Acupuncture

   b. Active wound care

   c. Osteopathic Manipulative

d. Home health procedures

137. A form of manual treatment applied by a physician to eliminate or alleviate somatic dysfunction and related disorders is?

   a. Acupuncture

   b. Active wound care

   c. Osteopathic Manipulative

   d. Home health procedures

138. _____ codes are used by non-physician health care professionals only to report services provided in a patient's residence?

   a. Acupuncture

   b. Active wound care

   c. Osteopathic Manipulative

   d. Home health procedures

139. Which of this is not a main section of the CPT-4?

   a. Surgery

   b. Radiology

   c. Medicine

   d. None of the above

140. Which of the following is a purpose of the CPT-4?

   a. To encourage the use of standard terms and descriptors to document procedures

   b. To provide basis for a computer oriented system to evaluate operative procedures

   c. To contribute basic information for statistical purposes

d. All of the above

141. The maximum amount of money that many third-party payors allow for a specific procedure or service is called?

   a. Maximum charge

   b. Third-party charge

   c. Allowed charge

   d. Authorized charge

142. Individual entitled to receive benefits from an insurance policy or government entitlement program offering healthcare benefits is?

   a. Beneficiary

   b. Benefiting participant

   c. Individual benefit

   d. Recipient

143. Payment method used by many managed care organization wherein a fixed amount of money is reimbursed to the provider for patients enrolled during a specific period of time is?

   a. Fixed payment

   b. Enrollment reimbursement

   c. Payment reimbursement

   d. Capitation

144. Health benefits program run by the department of veterans affairs that helps eligible beneficiaries pay the cost of specific healthcare services and supplies is?

a. CHAMPUS

b. CHUMPVA

c. CHAMPVA

d. Benefits for veteran affairs

145. A policy provision frequently found in medical insurance whereby the policyholder and the insurance company share the cost of covered losses in a specified ratio is?

a. Copayment

b. Co-insurance

c. Co-ratio

d. Commercial insurance

146. A sum of money that is paid at the time of medical service is?

a. Copayment

b. Co-insurance

c. Co-ratio

d. Commercial insurance

147. Plans that reimburse the insured for expenses resulting from illness or injury according to a specific fee schedule as outlined in the insurance policy on a fee-for-service basis is?

a. Copayment

b. Co-insurance

c. Co-ratio

d. Commercial insurance

148. Which of the following is also called subscriber?

   a. Beneficiary

   b. Benefiting participant

   c. Individual benefit

   d. Recipient

149. Which of this is sometimes called private insurance?

   a. Copayment

   b. Co-insurance

   c. Co-ratio

   d. Commercial insurance

150. Specific amounts of money a patient must pay out of pocket before the insurance carrier begins paying is?

   a. Copayment

   b. Out of pocket payment

   c. Initial payment

   d. Deductibles

151. The spouse, children and sometimes partner or other individuals designated by the insured who are covered under a healthcare plan is?

   a. Dependent

   b. Defendant

   c. Respondent

   d. Independent

152. Insurance that provides periodic payment to replace income when an insured person is unable to work as a result of illness, injury or disease is?

   a. Employment disability

   b. Disability income insurance

   c. Illness Insurance

   d. All of the above

153. A letter or statement from the insurance carrier describing what was paid, denied or reduced in payment is?

   a. Exclusion

   b. Explanation of benefit

   c. Explanation of Medicare Benefits

   d. Statement of Insurance

154. Limitations on an insurance contract for which benefits are not payable is?

   a. Exclusion

   b. Explanation of benefit

   c. Explanation of Medicare Benefits

   d. Insurance limitation

155. An established schedule of fees set for services performed by providers and paid by the patient?

   a. Scheduled fee

   b. Service performance fee

   c. Fee for service

d. All of the above

156. An organization that contracts with government to handle and dedicate insurance claims from medical facilities or providers of medical services or supplies is?

   a. Government medical organization

   b. Insurance organization

   c. Fiscal intermediary

   d. None of the above

157. The person responsible for paying a medical bill is called?

   a. Health insurance

   b. Guarantor

   c. Sponsor

   d. Medicare

158. _____ is a federal program administered by state governments to provide medical assistance to the needy?

   a. Medigap

   b. Advance Beneficiary

   c. Medicaid

   d. Medi-cal

159. _____ is a private insurance designed to help pay for those amounts that are typically the patient's responsibility under Medicare?

   a. Medigap

   b. Advance Beneficiary

c. Medicaid

d. Medi-cal

160. Protection against financial losses resulting from illness or injury?

   a. Financial insurance

   b. Health insurance

   c. Insurance protection

   d. All of the above

161. The periodic payment of a specific sum of money to an insurance company for which the insurer agrees to provide certain benefit is?

   a. Monthly payment

   b. Annual payment

   c. Quarterly payment

   d. Premium

162. Which of this is not a type of health insurance?

   a. Group insurance

   b. Individual insurance

   c. Medical savings account

   d. None of the above

163. _____ is a contract between a policyholder and an insurance carrier or a government program developed to reimburse the policyholder of all or most medical expenses?

   a. Policy Holder contract

   b. Insurance carrier contract

c. Health insurance

d. Medicare

164. Which of this is not a way an individual can obtain health insurance?

   a. Group Insurance

   b. Personal Insurance

   c. Pre-paid Health Plan

   d. Employee Insurance

165. When a group of employees and their dependents are insured under one (1) group policy issued to the employer it is called?

   a. Group Insurance

   b. Personal Insurance

   c. Pre-paid Health Plan

   d. Employee Insurance

166. The _____ is also known as a fee for service?

   a. Indemnity Insurance

   b. Managed Care Plans

   c. Preferred Provider Organization

   d. Point-of-Service plan

167. _____ is a managed care plan that gives beneficiaries the option of whom to see for services?

   a. Preferred Provider Plan

b. Managed Care Plans

c. Preferred Provider Organization

d. Point-of-Service plan

168. The type of plan where a patient may have where they can see providers outside their plan is known as?

   a. Preferred Provider Plan

   b. Managed Care Plans

   c. Preferred Provider Organization

   d. Point-of-Service plan

169. What method is used mostly in reference to fee for-service reimbursement?

   a. Relative Value Payment Schedules Method

   b. Medicare's Resource Based Relative Value Scale (RBRVS) Payment Schedule

   c. The Usual, Customary, and Reasonable

   d. Contracted Rate Method

170. _____ Involves the use of relative value scales which assign a relative weight to individual services according to the basis for the scale?

   a. Relative Value Payment Schedules Method

   b. Medicare's Resource Based Relative Value Scale (RBRVS) Payment Schedule

   c. The Usual, Customary, and Reasonable

   d. Contracted Rate Method

171. Which of this does the Physicians agree to provide services at a discount of their usual fee in return for a pool of existing patients?

   a. Contracted Rate with MCO

   b. Capitated Rates

   c. The Usual, Customary, and Reasonable

   d. Relative Value Payment Schedules Method

172. Medicare is available for the following categories of people except?

   a. Person who does not want to pay medical bill

   b. persons 65 years or older, retired on Social Security benefits

   c. those diagnosed with end-stage renal disease

   d. spouse of a person paying into the Social Security system

173. _____ is a document provided to a Medicare beneficiary by a provider prior to service being rendered letting the beneficiary know of his/her responsibility to pay if Medicare denies the claim?

   a. Medigap

   b. Advance Beneficiary

   c. Medicaid

   d. Medi-cal

174. Which of this is not a service offered by Medicaid?

   a. Outpatient hospital services

   b. Cosmetic procedures necessitated by an injury

   c. Family planning and supplies

d. None of the above

175. _____ is a state-required insurance plan, the coverage of which provides benefits to employees and their dependents for work related injury, illness or death?

   a. Employee Insurance
   b. Employer Insurance
   c. Workers Compensation
   d. State Insurance

176. _____ is a policy that covers losses to a third party caused by the insured, by an object owned by the insured, or on premises owned by the insured?

   a. Disability
   b. Liability
   c. Comprehensive
   d. Auto insurance

177. Which of this is not a type of plan covered under the TRICARE program

   a. Standard
   b. Active
   c. Extra
   d. Prime

178. Which of the plans covered under TRICARE does not have annual deductible?

   a. Standard
   b. Active
   c. Extra

d. Prime

179. Which of the plans covered under TRICARE is a health maintenance organization plan with a point-of-service option?

   a. Standard

   b. Active

   c. Extra

   d. Prime

180. Which of this was created to provide medical benefits to spouses and children of veterans with total, permanent service related disabilities or for surviving spouses and children of a veteran who died as a result of service related to disability?

   a. TRICARE

   b. CHAMPUS

   c. CHAMPVA

   d. All of the above

181. In the Medicare suffix status chart "A" means?

   a. Disabled Child

   b. Widow

   c. Disabled adult

   d. Wage earner

182. In the Medicare suffix status chart "D" means?

   a. Disabled Child

   b. Widow

c. Disabled adult

d. Wage earner

183. Which of the medicare parts is referred to as Supplementary Medical Insurance?

a. Part A

b. Part B

c. Part C

d. Part D

184. Which of the medicare parts is also called Hospital Insurance for the Aged and Disabled?

a. Part A

b. Part B

c. Part C

d. Part D

185. Amongst the terms used to describe the state of submitted forms "Dirty Claim" means?

a. Has all required fields accurately filled out, contains no deficiencies.

b. Contains errors or omissions

c. Requires investigation and needs further clarification

d. Contains complete, necessary information, but is incorrect or illogical in some way

186. Amongst the terms used to describe the state of submitted forms "Rejected Claim" means?

a. Has all required fields accurately filled out, contains no deficiencies.

b. Contains errors or omissions

c. Requires investigation and needs further clarification

d. Contains complete, necessary information, but is incorrect or illogical in some way

187. Amongst the terms used to describe the state of submitted forms "Invalid Claim" means?

   a. Has all required fields accurately filled out, contains no deficiencies.

   b. Contains errors or omissions

   c. Requires investigation and needs further clarification

   d. Contains complete, necessary information, but is incorrect or illogical in some way

188. _____ is a traditional method used by providers for submission of charges to insurance companies?

   a. Paper Claim

   b. Electronic Claim

   c. Clearinghouse

   d. Universal Claim Form

189. _____ is an entity that receives transmissions of claims from physicians' offices, separates the claims by carriers and performs software edits on each claim to check for errors?

   a. Paper Claim

   b. Electronic Claim

   c. Clearinghouse

   d. Universal Claim Form

190. Which of the following is not a basic billing and reimbursement steps?

   a. Calculate physician charges

   b. Transmit claims

   c. Verify insurance

   d. None of the above

191. The transmission of claims data either electronically or manually to third party payers or clearinghouses for processing is known as?

   a. Claims processing

   b. Claims adjudication

   c. Claims submission

   d. Claim Payment

192. _____ is when the third party payers and clearinghouses verify the information found in the submitted claims about the patient and provider?

   a. Claims processing

   b. Claims adjudication

   c. Claims submission

   d. Claim Payment

193. Any procedure or service reported on the insurance claim that is not listed in the payer's master benefit list is called?

   a. Unauthorized benefit

   b. Unlisted benefit

   c. Non-covered benefit

   d. Denied Benefit

194. A procedure or service provided without proper authorization or was not covered by a current authorization

   a. Unauthorized benefit

   b. Unlisted benefit

c. Non-covered benefit

d. Denied Benefit

195. _____ is when the provider agrees to accept what the insurance company approves as payment in full for the claim.

 a. Assignment of benefits.

 b. Accept assignment

 c. Insurance agreement

 d. Provider-insurance acceptance

196. A patient who receives treatment in the hospital clinic or physician's office and released within 23hrs is known as?

 a. Impatient

 b. Outpatient

 c. Hospital patient

 d. Less than a day patient

197. A patient that is admitted to the hospital with the expectation that the patient will stay for a period of 24 hours or more is called?

 a. Impatient

 b. Outpatient

 c. Hospital patient

 d. More than a day patient

198. A service performed by a physician whose opinion or advice is requested by another physician in the evaluation or treatment of a patient's illness or suspected problem is called?

a. Advisory

b. Consultation

c. Counseling

d. Conferencing

199. A claim that is missing information and is returned to the provider for correction and resubmission is called?

a. Incorrect claim

b. Missing claim

c. Resubmission claim

d. Incomplete claim

200. _____ is also called invalid claim?

a. Incorrect claim

b. Missing claim

c. Resubmission claim

d. Incomplete claim

201. Which of this is a section in which the CMS-1500 is divided into?

a. Address of the insurance carrier

b. Physician's information

c. Patient Information

d. All of the above

202. Claims without significant errors of any type is called?

a. Non error claim

b. Clean claim

c. Semi-clean claim

d. Dirty claim

203. Inaccurate or incomplete insurance claim returned for information and correction is?

   a. Correct claim

   b. Inaccurate claim

   c. Dingy claim

   d. Partial claim

204. _____ is referred to as the path left by electronic transaction when it has been completed?

   a. Completed trail

   b. Audit trail

   c. Tickler trail

   d. None of the above

205. A record of the charges and payment posted on an account is called?

   a. Accounts receivable ledger

   b. Account balance

   c. Account record

   d. Payment record

206. An entry on an account constituting an addition to a revenue, net worth or liability account is?

   a. Debit

   b. Credit

   c. Liability

   d. Revenue

207. An entry on an account constituting an addition to an expense or asset account or a deduction from a revenue, a net worth, or a liability account is?

   a. Debit

   b. Credit

   c. Liability

   d. Revenue

208. Funds paid out is called?

   a. Disbursement

   b. Reimbursement

   c. Repay

   d. Refund

209. An organization under contract to the government as well as some private plans to act as financial representatives in handling insurance claims from providers of healthcare is called?

   a. Financial representatives

   b. Insurance provider

   c. Fiscal agent

d. Government financial agent

210. _____ is also referred to as fiscal intermediary?

   a. Financial representatives

   b. Insurance provider

   c. Fiscal agent

   d. Government financial agent

211. _____ is also called a write-it-once system?

   a. Posting

   b. Pegboard system

   c. Payables

   d. Premium

212. _____ is the consideration paid for a contract of insurance?

   a. Posting

   b. Pegboard system

   c. Payables

   d. Premium

213. A superiority or excess in number of quantity is?

   a. Preponderance

   b. Superior quantity

   c. Excess quantity

   d. None of the above

214. Amount paid on patient accounts is?

a. Receivables

b. Payment

c. Receipts

d. Third-party payor

215. Total monies received on account is?

a. Receivables

b. Payment

c. Receipts

d. Third-party payor

216. A method of accurately tracking patient accounts that allows the figure to be proved accurate through mathematic formulas is?

a. Posting

b. Pegboard system

c. Payables

d. Audit Trail

217. Most insurance plans base their payment of UCR fees, the "U" here means?

a. Unilateral

b. Union

c. Usual

d. Under

218. Most insurance plans base their payment of UCR fees, the "R" here means?

a. Rights

166

b. Reliance

c. Reliable

d. Reasonable

219. The slips that are attached to charts while the patient is in the office, usually for billing purpose is called?

   a. Billing slip

   b. In office slip

   c. Chart slip

   d. Encounter forms

220. When a patient has paid in advance or there has been an overpayment or duplicate payment it is called?

   a. Overpayment

   b. Debit balances

   c. Credit balances

   d. Advanced payment

221. Which of this is not a type of check?

   a. Certified check

   b. Limited check

   c. Money Order

   d. None of the above

222. Network of banks that exchange checks with one another is called?

   a. Banks exchange

   b. Check exchange

c. Clearinghouses

d. None of the above

223. When a mistake or an error is made on a check what should you do?

   a. Cross it out

   b. Rewrite on the error

   c. Write the word void on the check

   d. All of the above

224. Which of this is not a type of endorsement?

   a. Blank endorsement

   b. Limited endorsement

   c. Special endorsement

   d. Qualified endorsement

225. Which of this type of endorsement does the payee signs his name and makes the check payable to the bearer?

   a. Blank endorsement

   b. Limited endorsement

   c. Special endorsement

   d. Qualified endorsement

226. A person who signs his name on the back of a check for the purpose of transferring title to another person is called?

   a. Imposer

   b. Endorser

c. Indorser

d. Transfer of check

227. The process of providing that a bank statement and checkbook balance are in agreement is called?

   a. Reconciliation

   b. Balancing

   c. Check bank balancing

   d. All of the above

228. The method of accounting in which income is recorded when earned and expenses are recorded when incurred is?

   a. Balance sheet

   b. Account receivable

   c. Accrual basis of accounting

   d. Trial balance

229. A method of checking the accuracy of accounts is?

   a. Balance sheet

   b. Account receivable

   c. Accrual basis of accounting

   d. Trial balance

230. A financial statement for a specific date that shows the total assets, liabilities and capital of the business is called?

   a. Balance sheet

   b. Cash flow statement

c. Statement of income and expense

d. Disbursement Journal

231. A financial summary for a specific period that shows the beginning balance on hand, the receipts and disbursements during the period and the balance on hand at the end of the period is called?

    a. Balance sheet

    b. Cash flow statement

    c. Statement of income and expense

    d. Disbursement Journal

232. A summary of accounts paid out is called?

    a. Accounts payable

    b. Cash flow statement

    c. Statement of income and expense

    d. Disbursement Journal

233. Which of the following is not a kind of financial record?

    a. Daily Journal

    b. Checkbook

    c. Income slip

    d. Petty cash record

234. _____ is the oldest and simplest book keeping system?

   a. Double-Entry

   b. Single-Entry

   c. Write-it-once system

   d. Pegboard system

235. Which of this is not a function of a medical office manager?

   a. Recruiting new employees

   b. Planning staff meetings

   c. Dismissing employees

   d. None of the above

236. Which of this is not a type of leader?

   a. Transactional

   b. Transnational

   c. Transformational

   d. Charismatic

237. _____ leader is innovative and able to bring about change in an organization?

   a. Transactional

   b. Transnational

   c. Transformational

   d. Charismatic

238. _____ is the ability to influence employees so that they carry out their directives?

    a. Influence

    b. Skill

    c. Power

    d. Affluence

239. _____ is a tool designed to inform employees about the duties they are expected to perform?

    a. Employee Handbook

    b. Employee manual

    c. Job description

    d. Policy manual

240. A series of executive position in order of authority is?

    a. Executive position

    b. Chain of command

    c. Organizational structure

    d. Line of management

241. The process or technique of promoting, selling and distributing a product or service is called?

   a. Promotion

   b. Marketing

   c. Outreach

   d. Target Market

242. The process of using marketing and education strategies to reach and involve diverse audiences through the use of key messages and effective programs is?

   a. Promotion

   b. Marketing

   c. Outreach

   d. Target Market

243. A special group of individuals towards whom the marketing plan is focused is?

   a. Promotion

   b. Marketing

   c. Outreach

   d. Representing

244. Which of the following is not one of the 4 "p's" of marketing?

   a. Product

   b. Price

   c. Placement

   d. Plan

245. An accounting period of 12 months is?

   a. Annual year

   b. Fiscal year

   c. 1 year

   d. None of the above

246. Traditional health insurance plans that pay for all or a share of the cost of covered services, regardless of which physician, hospital or other healthcare provider is used is called?

   a. Indemnity

   b. Service benefit plan

   c. UCR Fee

   d. Resource-based relative value scale

247. Which of this is not a health care provider?

   a. Managed care plans

   b. Blue Cross

   c. Commercial insurance

   d. None of the above

248. Which of this is not a model of managed care?

   a. HMO

   b. PPO

   c. MCO

   d. None of the above

249. A fee schedule designed to provide national uniform payment of medicare benefits after being adjusted to reflect the differences in practice cost across geographic areas is called?

   a. Indemnity

   b. Service benefit plan

   c. UCR Fee

   d. Resource-based relative value scale

250. A process required by some insurance carriers where the provider obtains permission to perform certain procedures or services or refer a patient to a specialist is called?

   a. Pre-certification

   b. Pre-determination

   c. Pre-authorization

   d. Pre-verification

MA Test 2	
1	D
2	B
3	B
4	C
5	B
6	C
7	A
8	C
9	D
10	A
11	B
12	A
13	B
14	D
15	D
16	B
17	D
18	C
19	A
20	A
21	D
22	C
23	D
24	B
25	B
26	C
27	B
28	A
29	B
30	D
31	B
32	B
33	C
34	C
35	A
36	B
37	D
38	A
39	A
40	B

41	C
42	C
43	D
44	A
45	B
46	A
47	C
48	C
49	A
50	D
51	B
52	A
53	A
54	C
55	C
56	C
57	C
58	B
59	D
60	C
61	C
62	D
63	B
64	B
65	D
66	B
67	D
68	D
69	A
70	B
71	D
72	C
73	D
74	A
75	D
76	C
77	B
78	D
79	A
80	A
81	C
82	C
83	A
84	C

85	D
86	C
87	C
88	B
89	B
90	A
91	B
92	D
93	C
94	B
95	C
96	C
97	D
98	B
99	B
100	A
101	D
102	C
103	B
104	C
105	C
106	D
107	B
108	A
109	A
110	B
111	C
112	A
113	A
114	D
115	B
116	B
117	C
118	C
119	B
120	**D**
121	C
122	A
123	C
124	D
125	A
126	D
127	B

128	D
129	A
130	B
131	B
132	A
133	C
134	A
135	B
136	A
137	C
138	D
139	D
140	D
141	C
142	A
143	D
144	C
145	B
146	A
147	D
148	A
149	D
150	D
151	A
152	B
153	B
154	A
155	C
156	C
157	B
158	C
159	A
160	A
161	D
162	D
163	C
164	D
165	A
166	A
167	D
168	A
169	C
170	A
171	A

172	A
173	B
174	D
175	C
176	B
177	B
178	D
179	D
180	C
181	D
182	B
183	B
184	A
185	B
186	C
187	D
188	A
189	C
190	D
191	C
192	A
193	C
194	A
195	B
196	B
197	A
198	B
199	D
200	D
201	D
202	B
203	C
204	B
205	A
206	B
207	A
208	A
209	C
210	C
211	B
212	D
213	A
214	C

215	A
216	B
217	C
218	D
219	D
220	C
221	D
222	C
223	C
224	B
225	A
226	B
227	A
228	C
229	D
230	A
231	B
232	D
233	C
234	B
235	D
236	B
237	C
238	C
239	C
240	B
241	B
242	C
243	D
244	D
245	B
246	A
247	D
248	C
249	D
250	C

Made in the USA
Columbia, SC
19 January 2019